Sadie Bug

Written and Illustrated by
Elizabeth Brandon

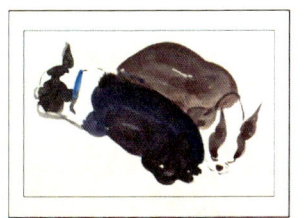

Bug-a-Muffin Books

Copyright © 2011 by Elizabeth Brandon.
All rights reserved.

ISBN: 978-0-615-44813-8
Library of Congress Catalog Number: 2011911866

Sadie Bug is available from Amazon, Barnes and Noble
and other fine booksellers.

Autographed copies through www.elizabethbrandon.com

Book Design by Janice Phelps Williams

To Katie and James with love and imagination

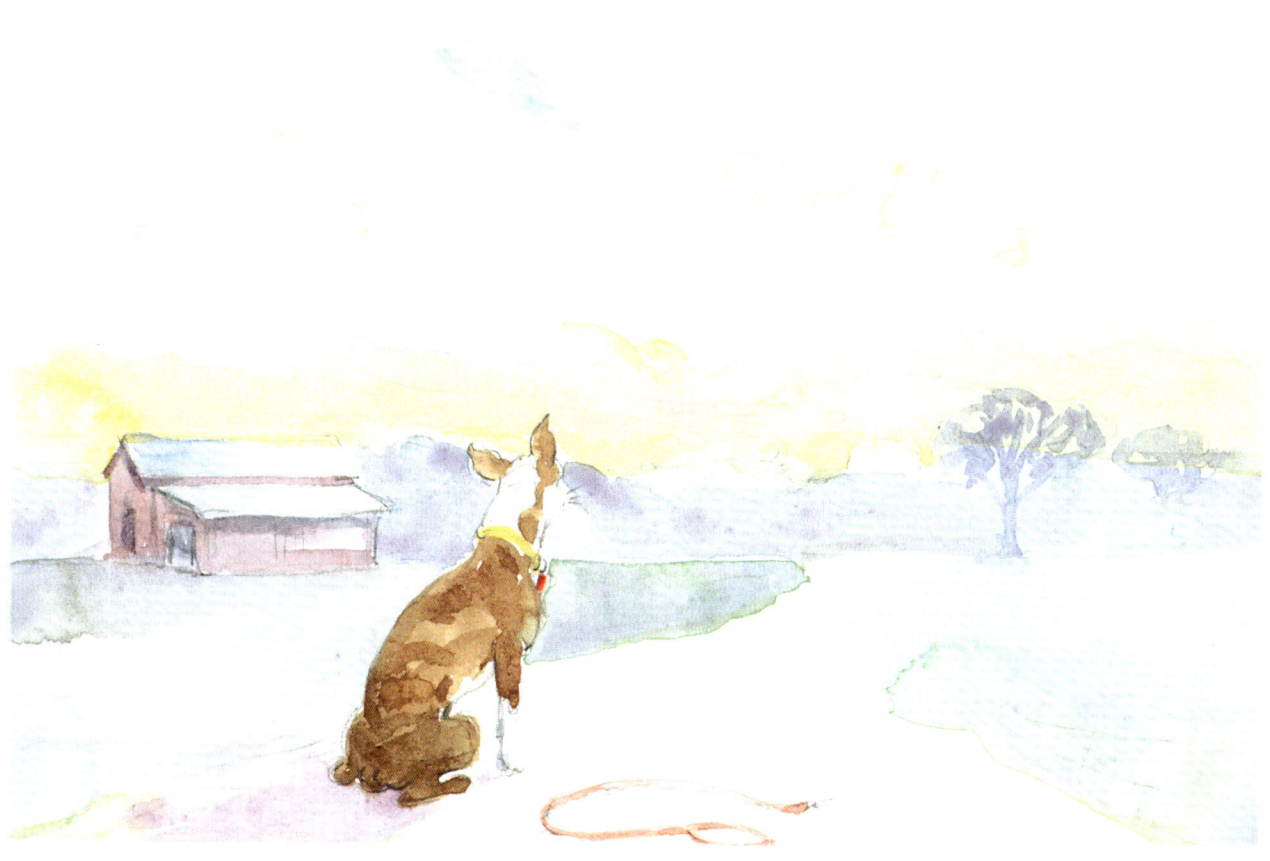

Salutations to the sun
To the awakening light within
To the dawning of higher consciousness
In all dogs, children, and parents.

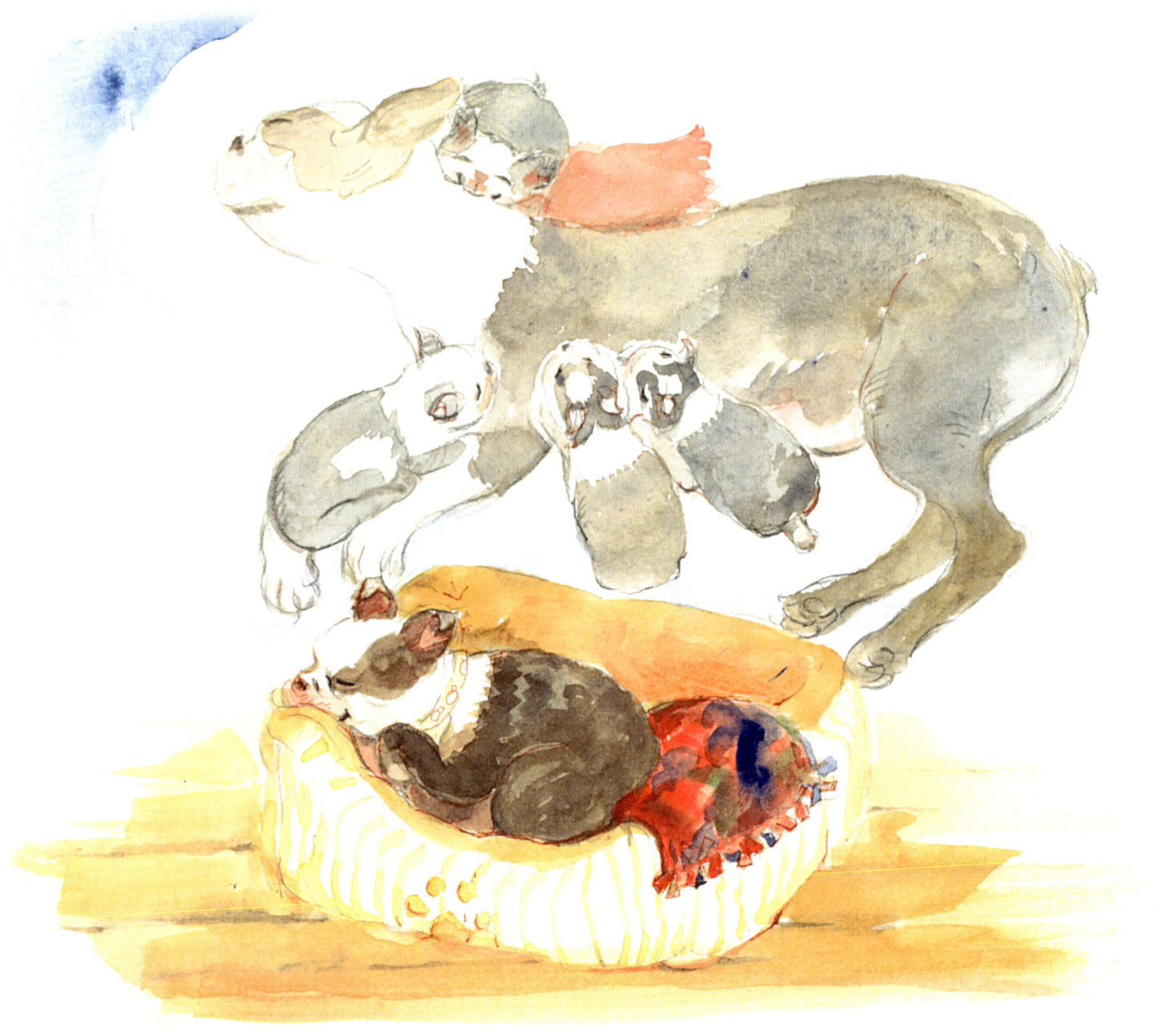

Sadie was asleep, having the most wonderful dream possible.

Suddenly, she awoke to a strange whistling sound of a teapot, that grew louder and louder. When she opened her eyes, she remembered she was in her own snuggly bed after a long day's journey.

Earlier, while she was riding in a car, Sadie woke up to a smiling face.

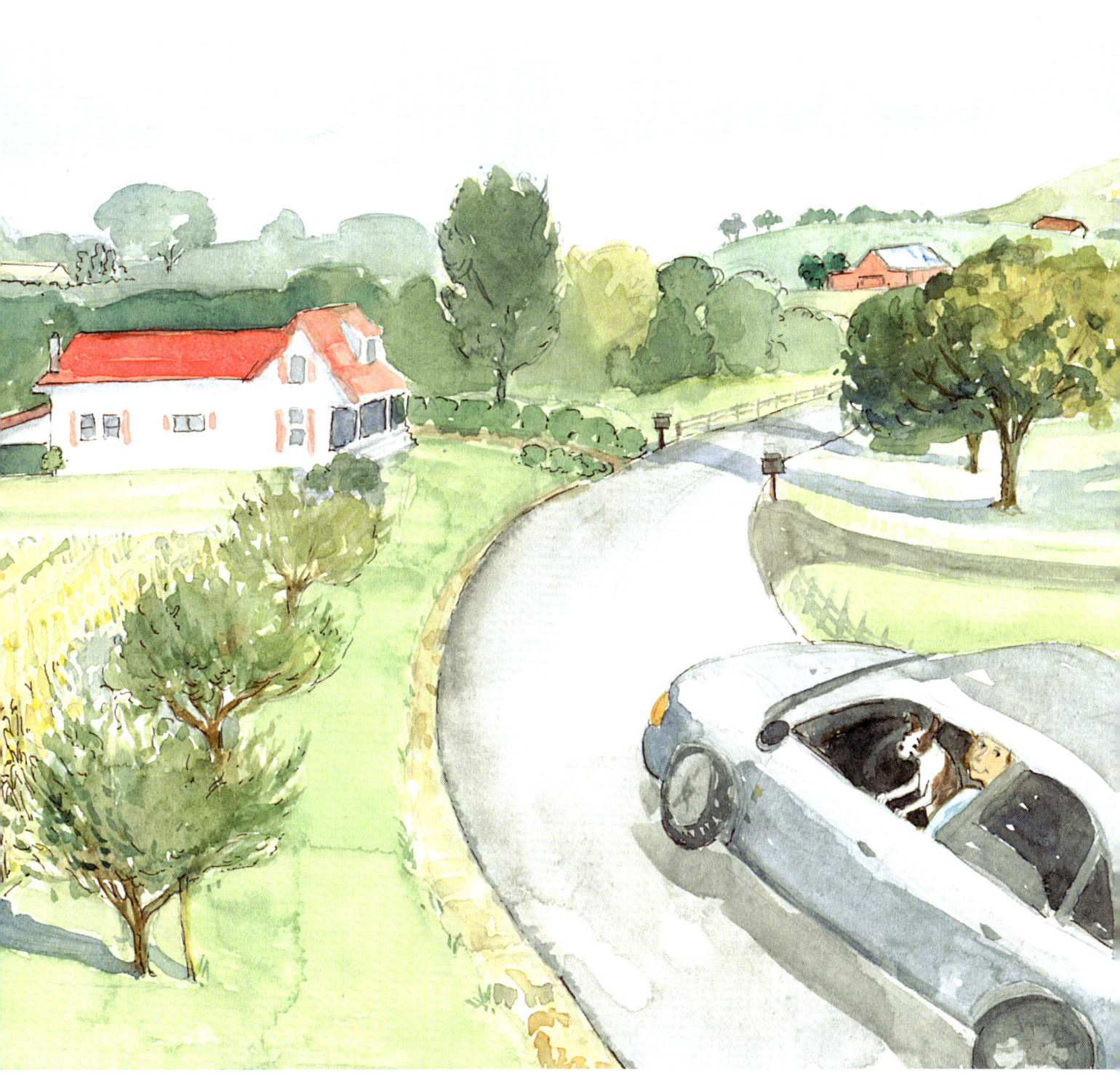

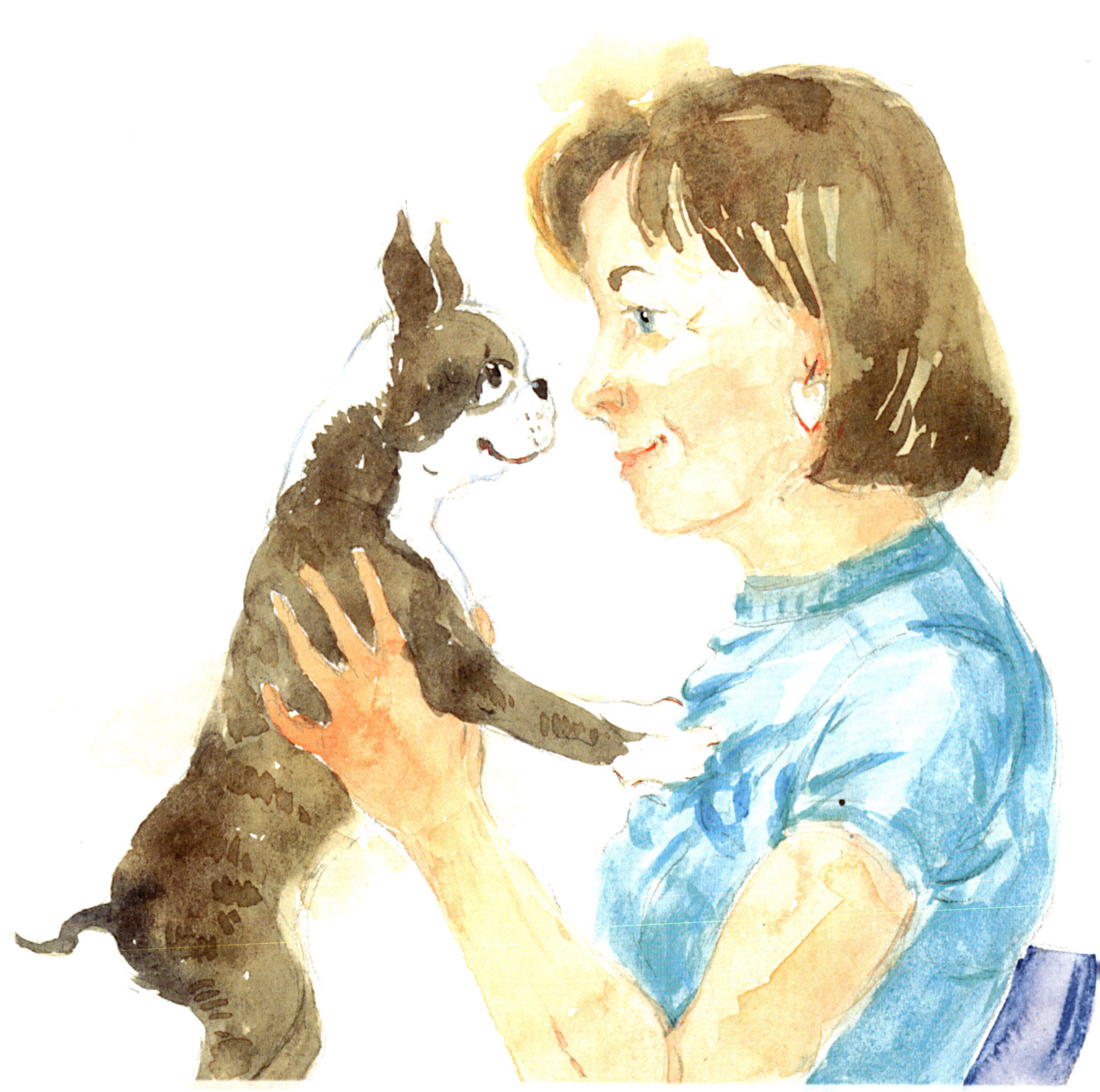

Her new mom picked her up tenderly and put her face right up to Sadie's wet nose. Little Sadie was happy to cuddle up in this warm, cozy lap and felt safe next to her body.

But her curiosity drew her attention to the world outside so she quickly jumped up to look outside the car window.

Where was she going?

Young Sadie had not seen much of the world and this place was new. She was happy, but also felt anxious. There was a small tug at her heart.

As they drove up the driveway, Sadie saw a big, beautiful, grassy yard.

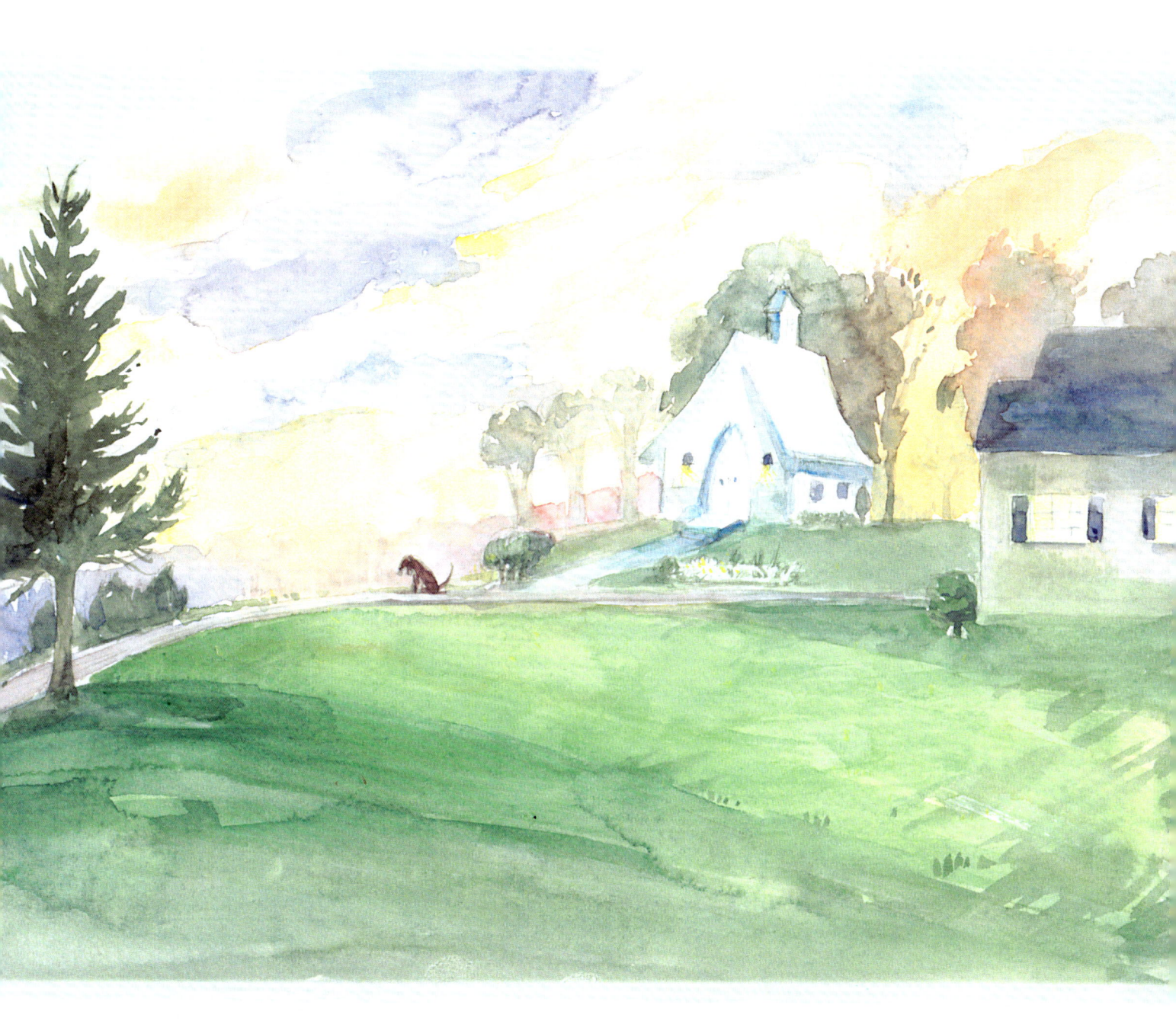

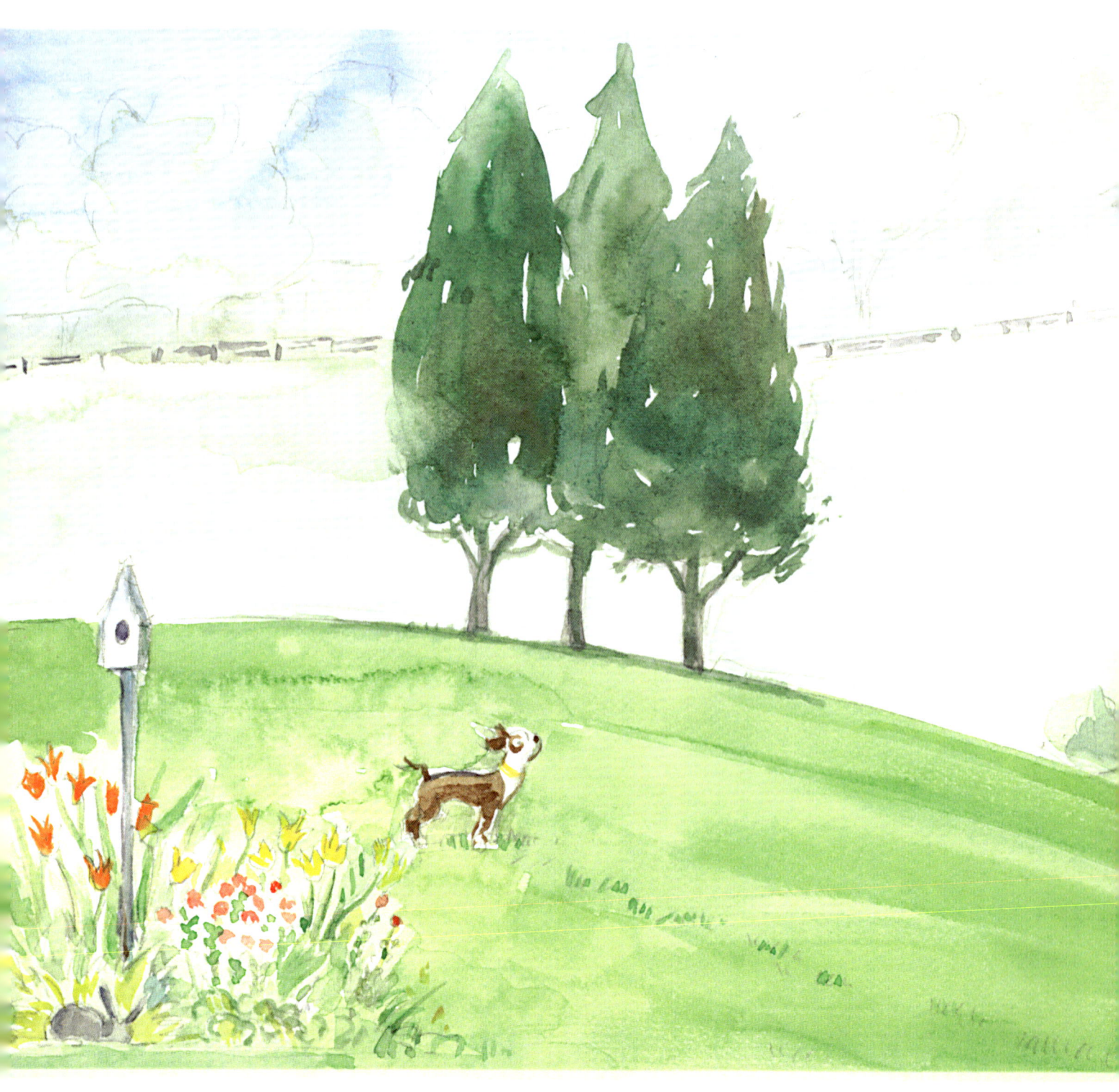

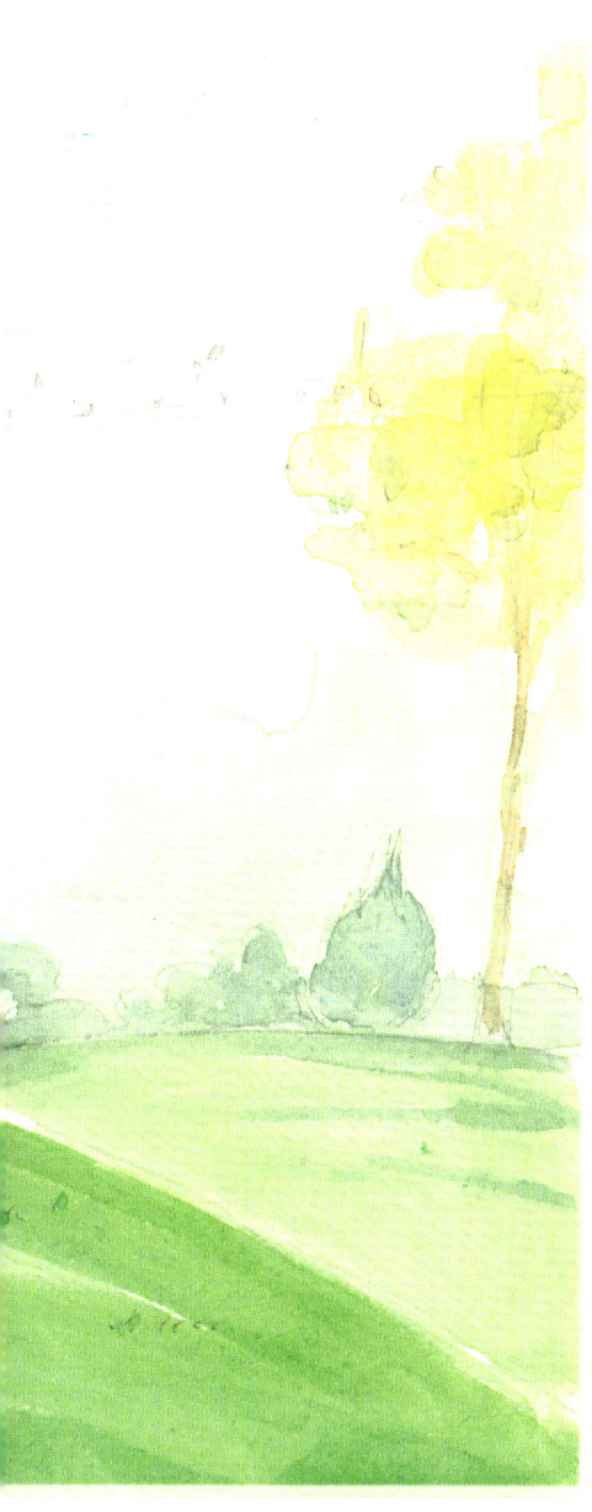

"Wow," she thought.
"I can run all over
this yard!"

This is what Sadie remembered as she woke in a new bed and smelled strange smells. She was feeling just a little bit lonely. Before she could feel alone any longer, her mom scooped her up and gave Sadie gentle hugs. She talked to Sadie about her new home. Sadie's uneasiness quickly melted into curiosity and a hungry tummy.

Breakfast was perfect, just like she liked it. This time she could have all the food to herself, with no sharing. That was nice.

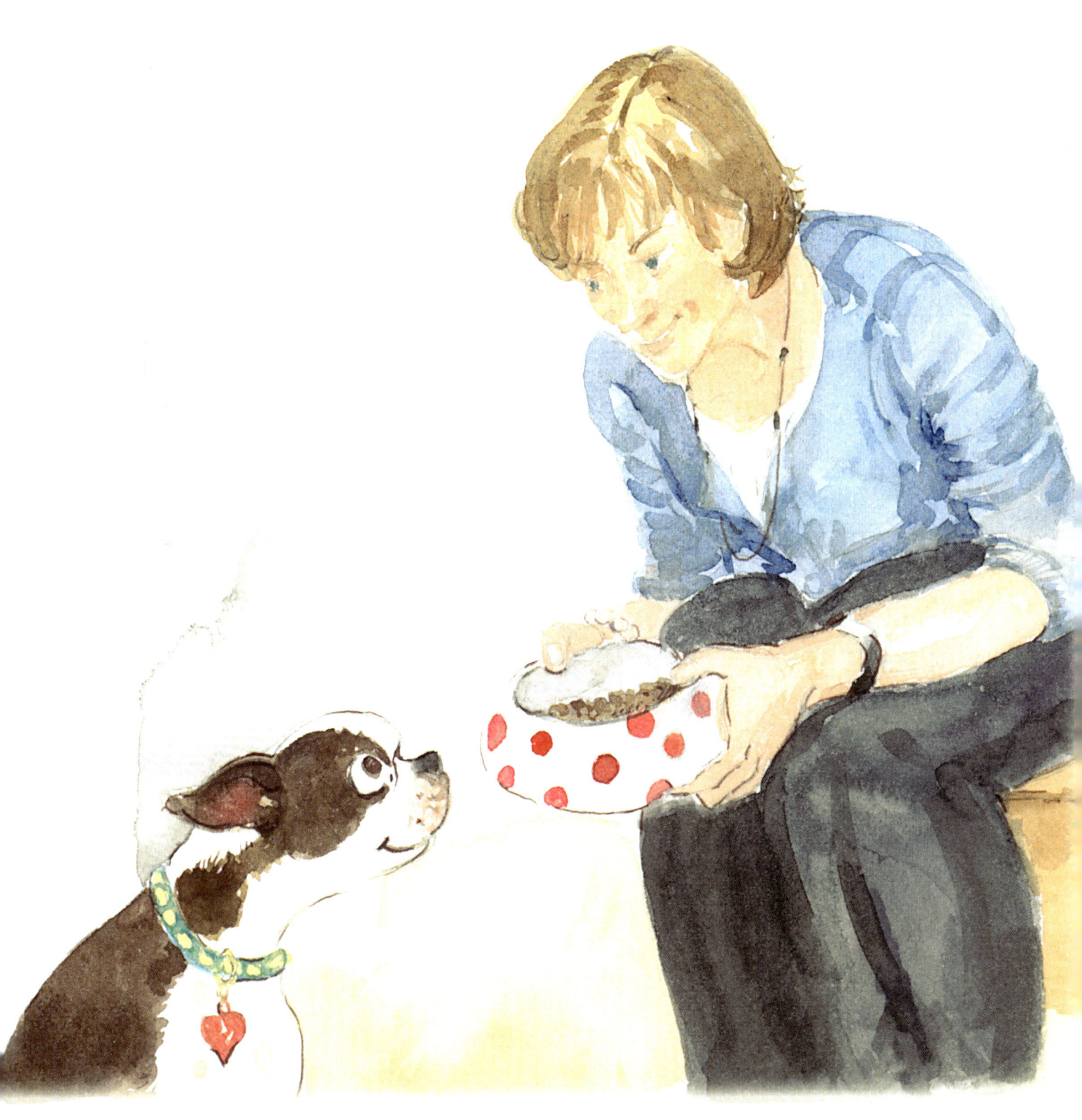

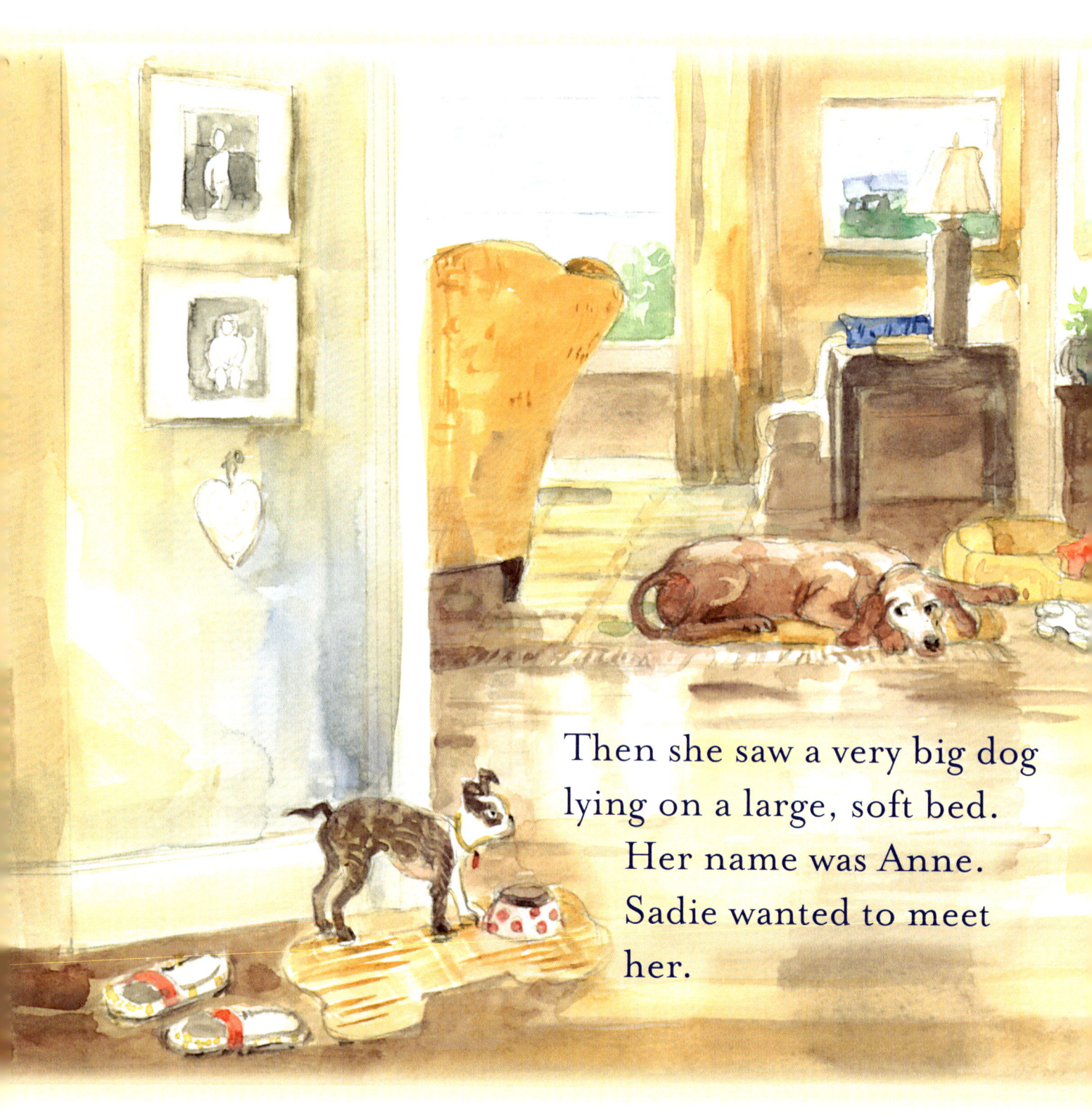

Then she saw a very big dog lying on a large, soft bed. Her name was Anne. Sadie wanted to meet her.

Sadie carefully and slowly inched her way to Anne's bedside. "Anne might be a pretty good friend," thought Sadie…

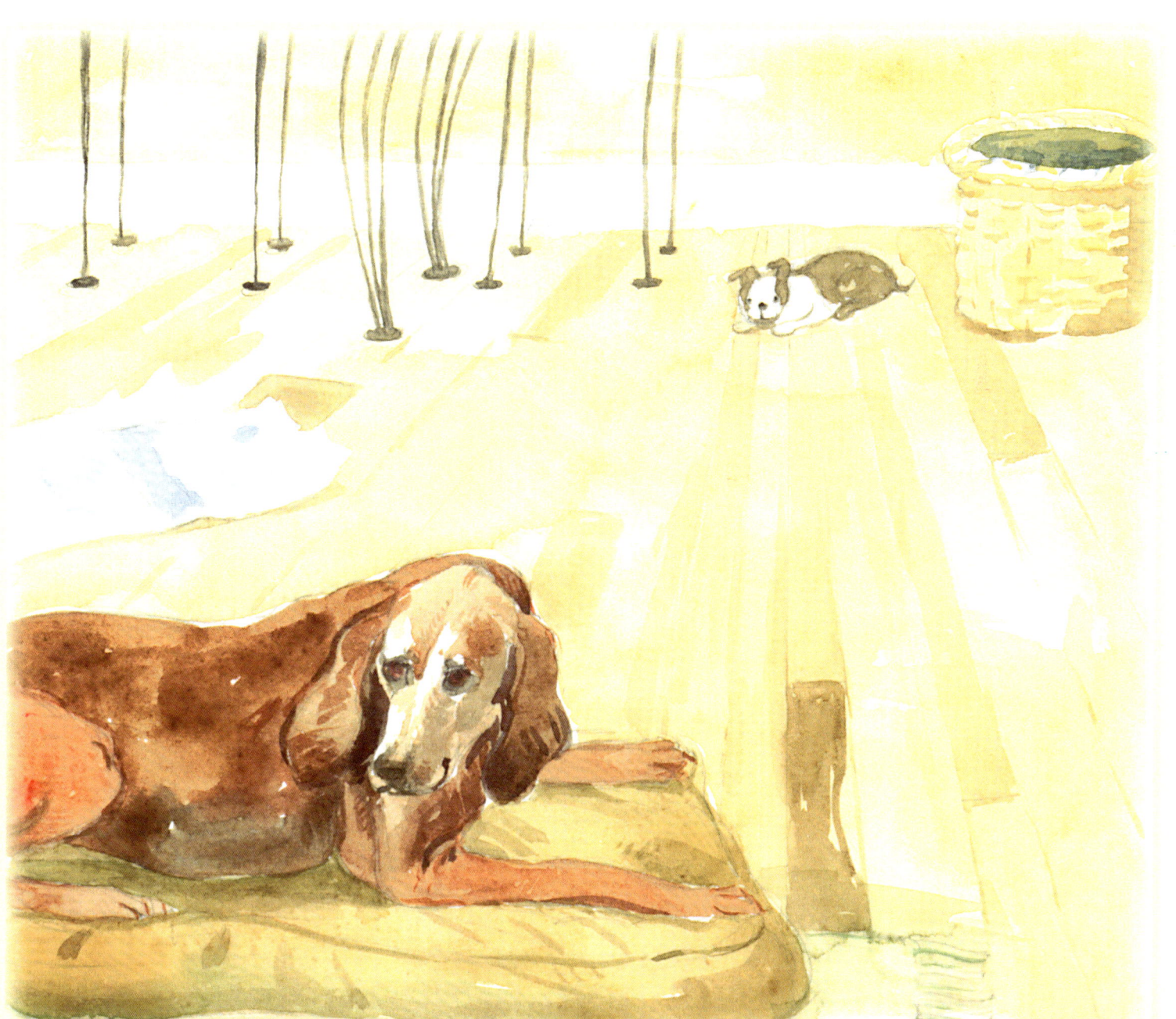

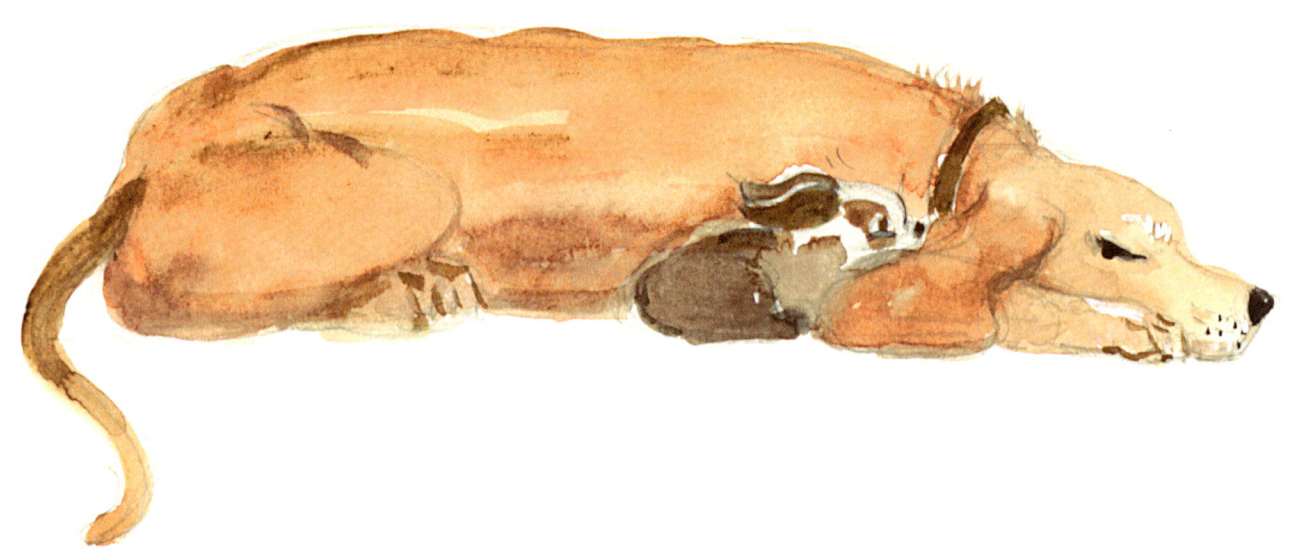

as she nestled next to Anne's long, soft ears.

After her tasty breakfast and a sweet, short puppy nap, Sadie ran to the door, wagging her tail to show she wanted to go outside. Maybe, they could find her a playmate out in the big yard. Anne was a very old dog, and Sadie longed to play with someone like herself. She wanted to tumble in the grass. Outside, Sadie saw something move in the tall grass.

She bravely ran over to see what it was. Sadie looked over the gentle hill and saw an enormous turkey. She thought it was awesome!

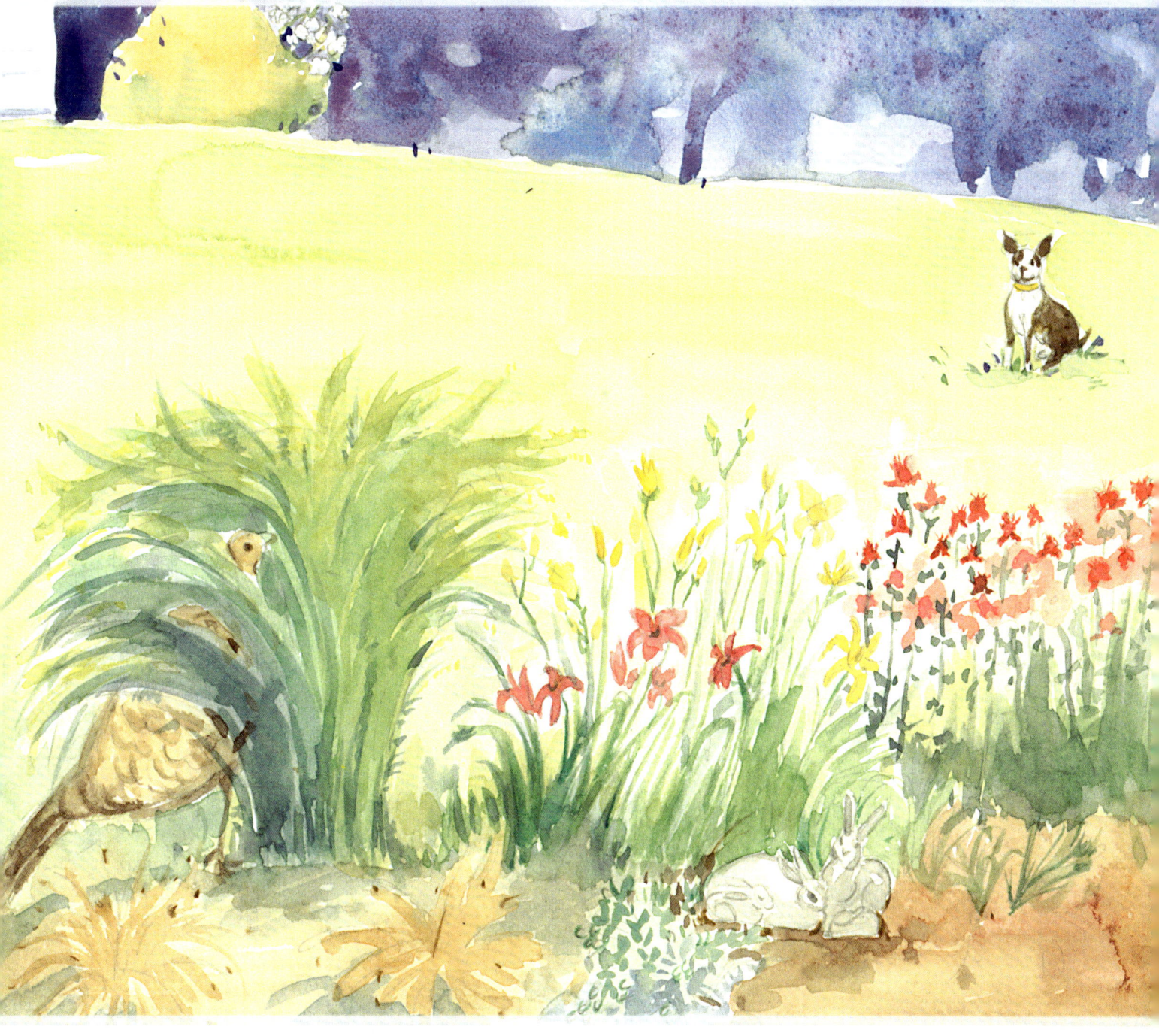

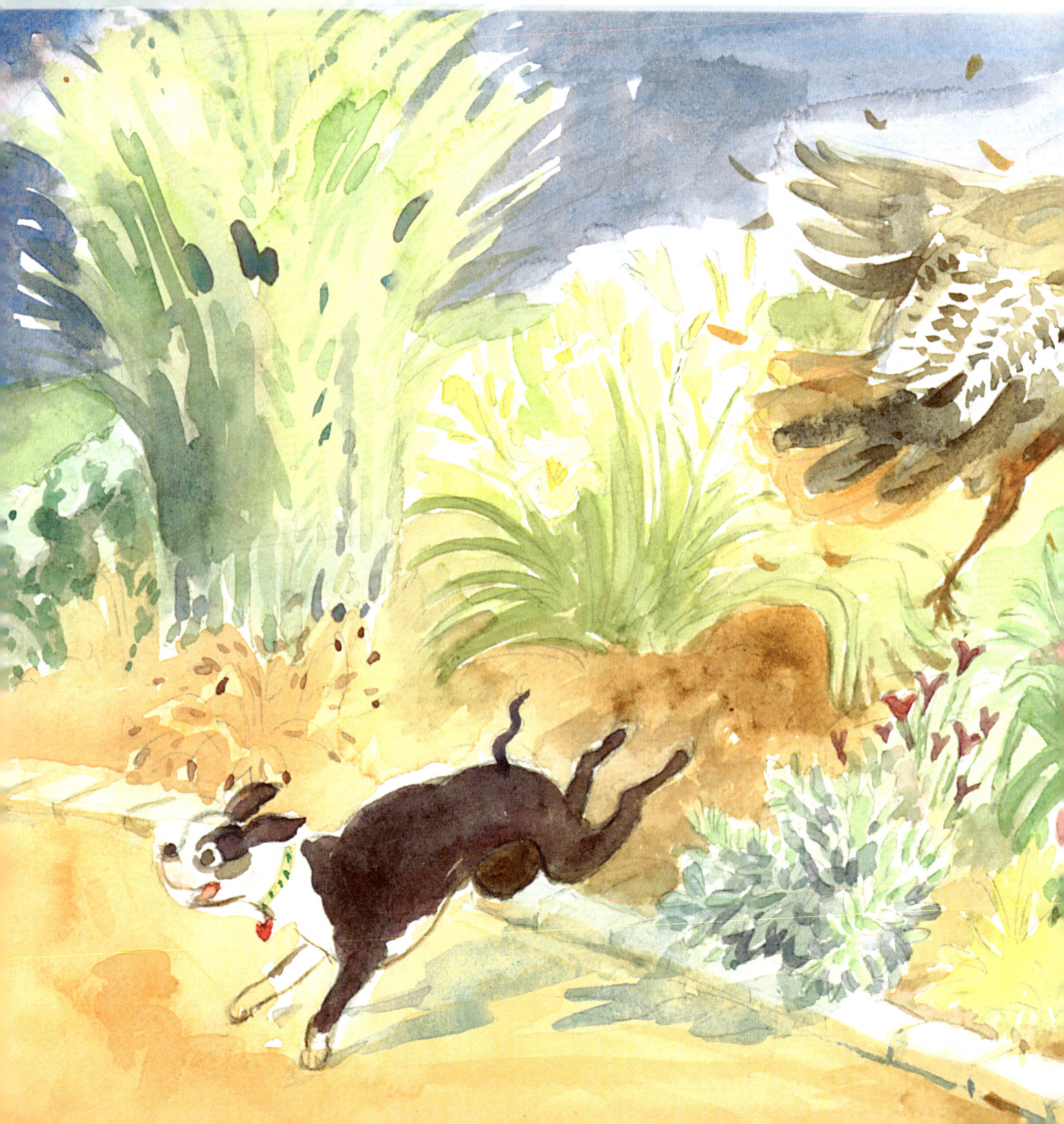

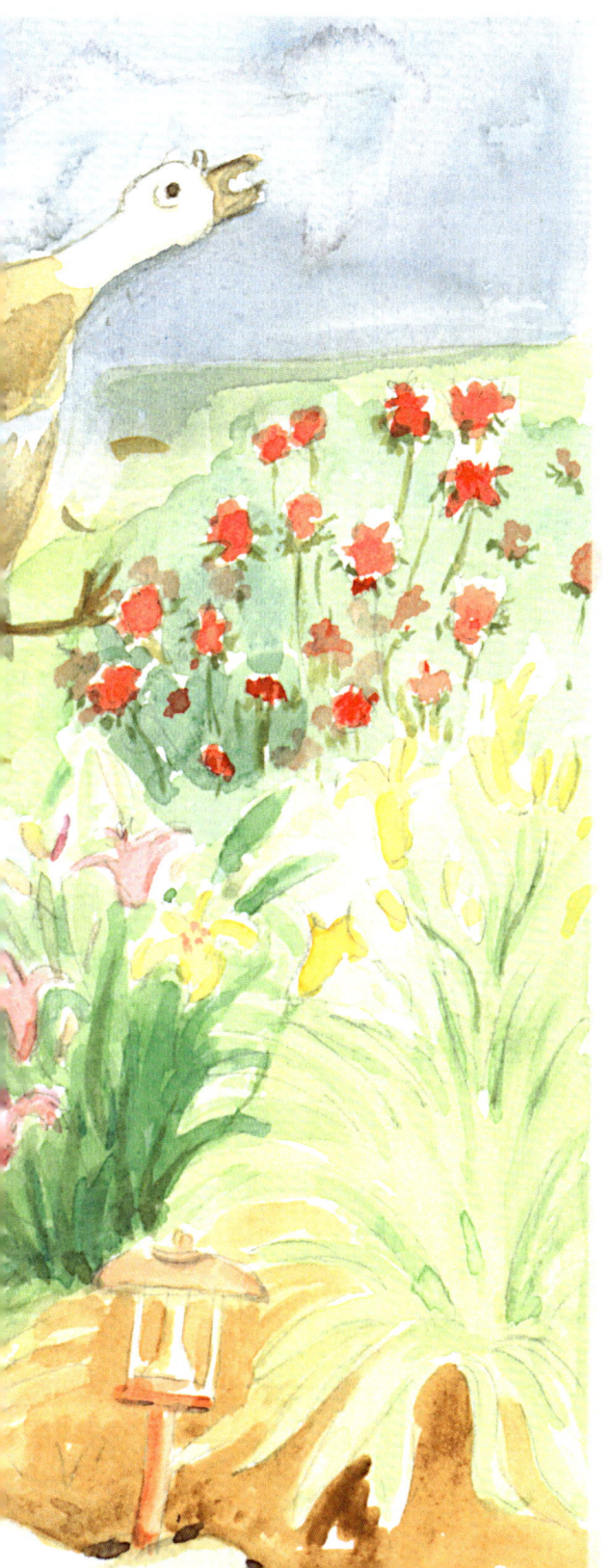

But only from a distance!

Sadie heard her name being called. She ran to her mom to get a tasty treat and come inside.

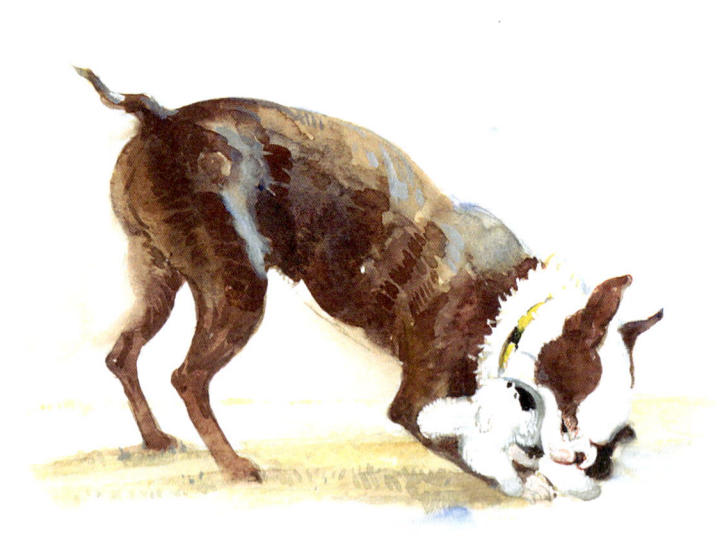

As she lay in a corner of her own special bed she saw something interesting. She decided to run over to see it. This funny looking creature didn't run away. Sadie barked a little to start a game. It made a noise too and that was great. It sort of looked like Sadie!! But, she had never heard *MOOO, MOOO, MOOO,* and she began to get excited about having a playful friend.

It didn't take long before Sadie knew she would have to do all the work herself to have fun. Her toy was new and cute, but it didn't make her feel happy for long. She needed something else to tumble around with in a longer, better way.

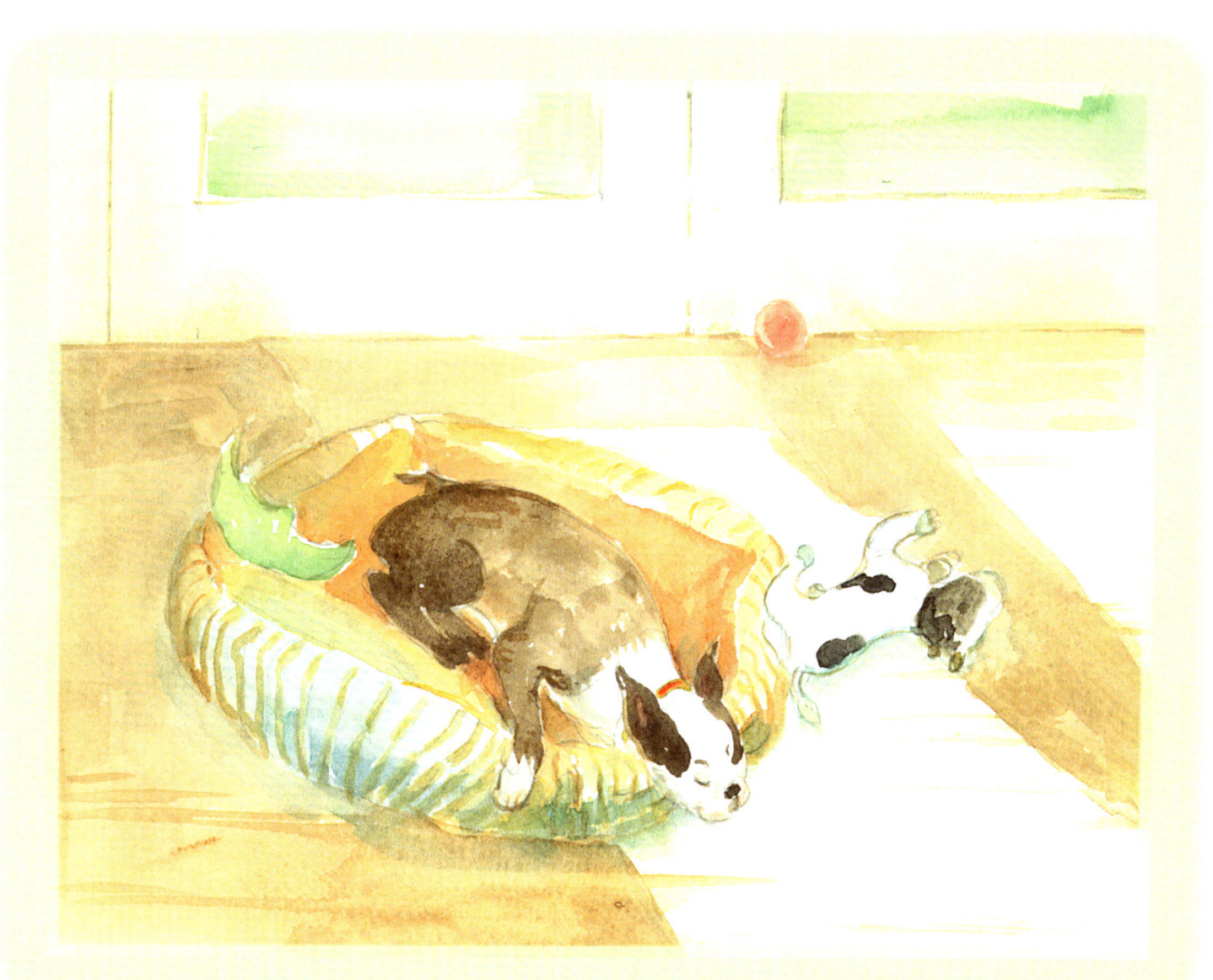

"Sadie Bug!" she heard her mom call. Her mom took Sadie by her side for a stroll down a country lane. Sadie's little eyes immediately saw some possible playmates. She unexpectedly pulled loose with her leash and slid under the fence. Sadie bounded across the field with glee and ran right into the middle of some really large creatures.

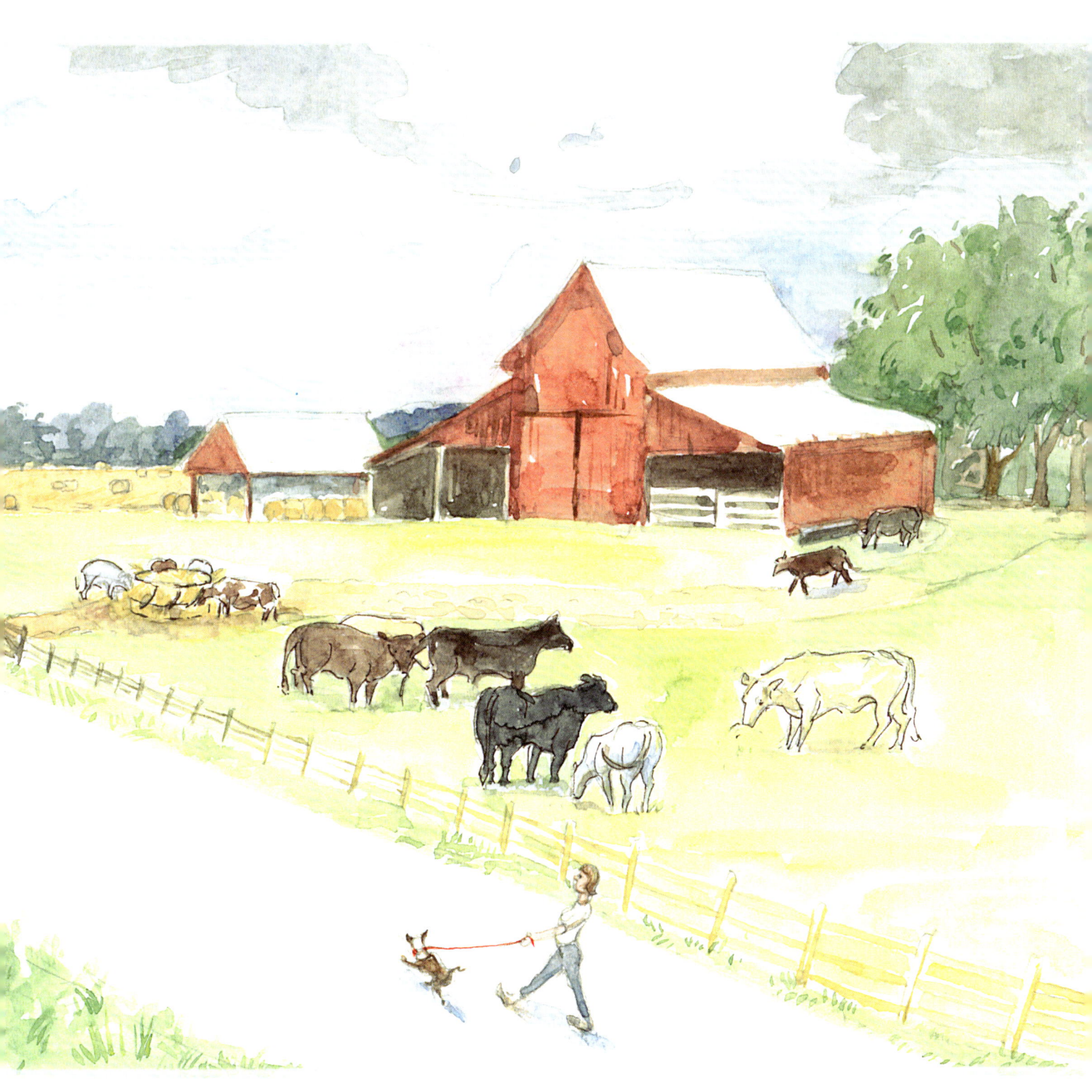

Sadie barked and jumped with excitement! But the big black-and-white animals just chewed and stood way too still for little Sadie. They couldn't understand what she was barking about and didn't want to play with her. A little disappointed, Sadie quietly walked back to her mom and together they continued their sunny day walk.

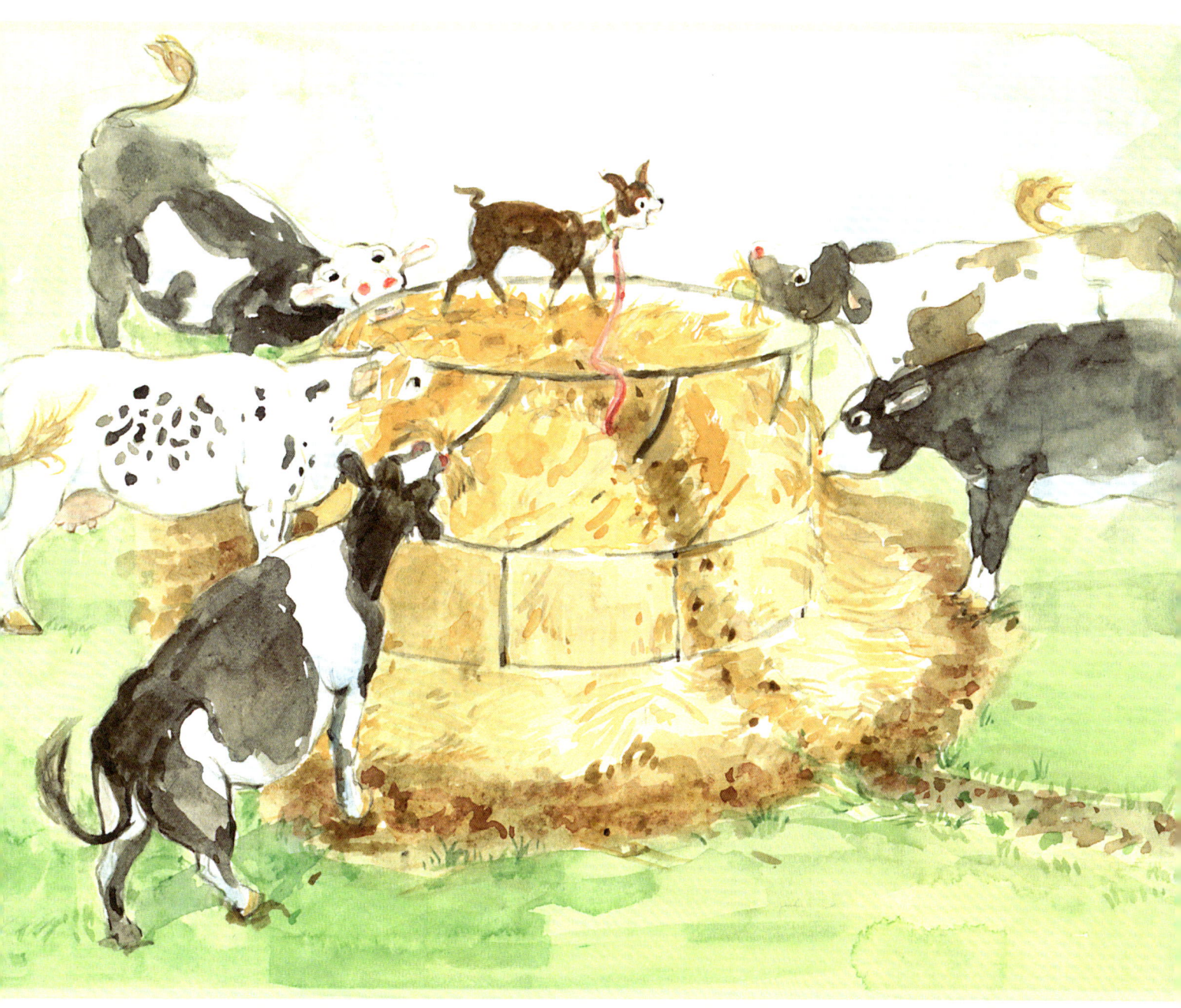

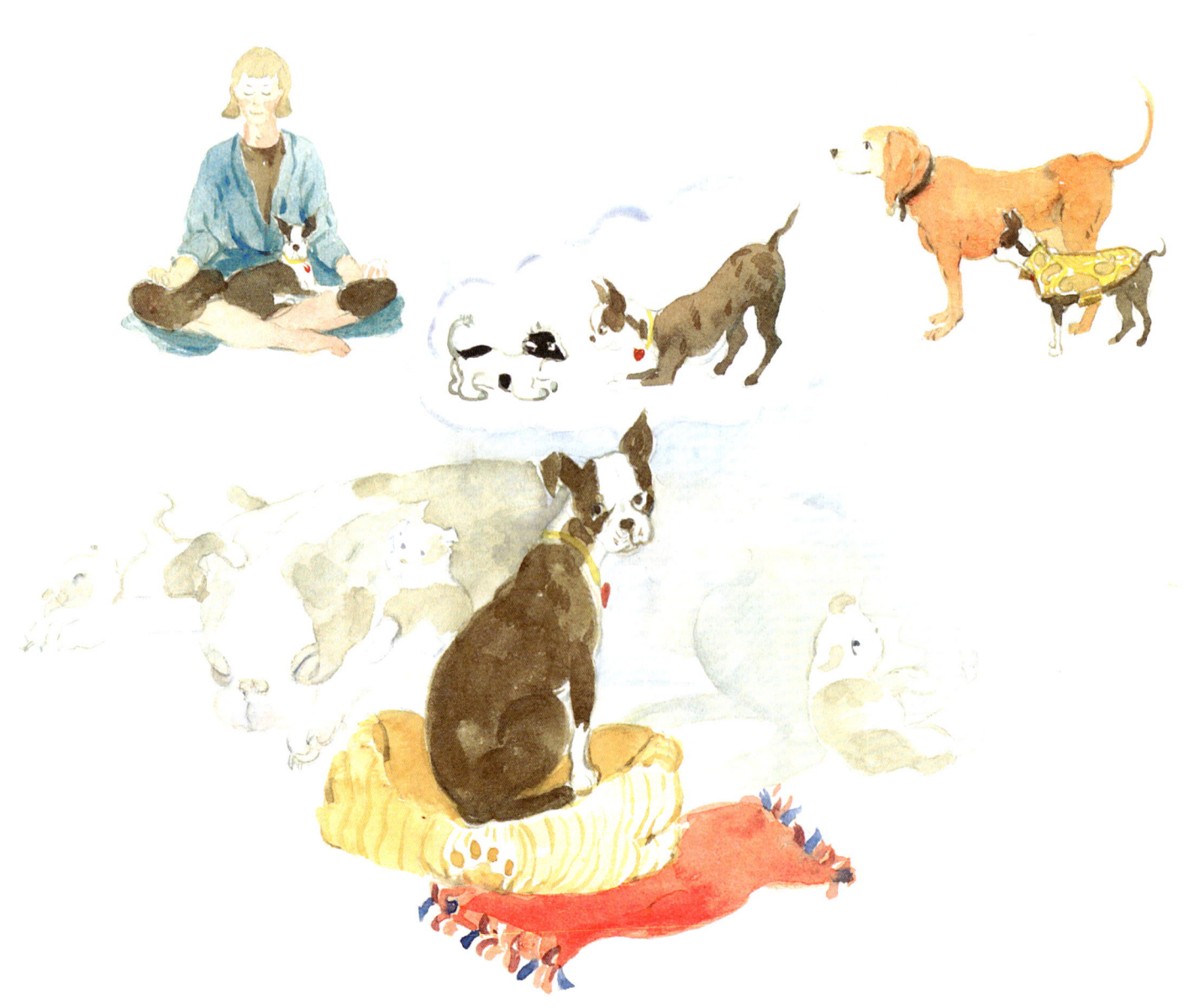

Back at home, Sadie Bug was thinking about her new mom, a funny toy, big dog Anne, and really strange animals who like to eat. Yet, she still dreamed to be with someone more like herself. Sadie again looked for something fun to do and someone special to do it with. She found her mom playing yoga ball. Her mom was really trying to play with her like a real best friend and it was pretty fun…for a while.

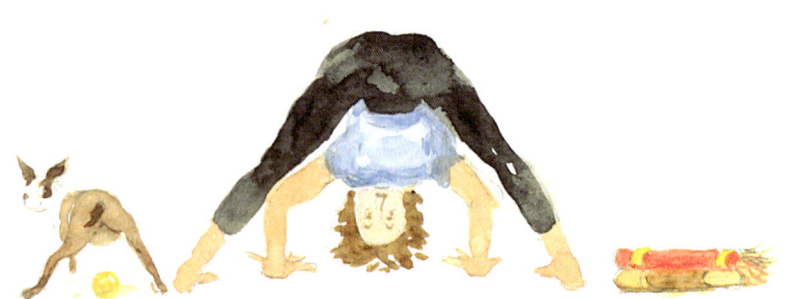
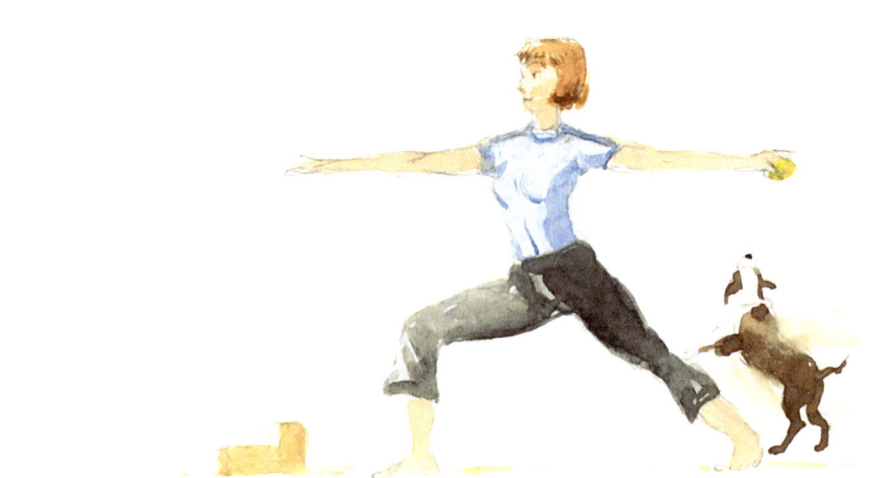
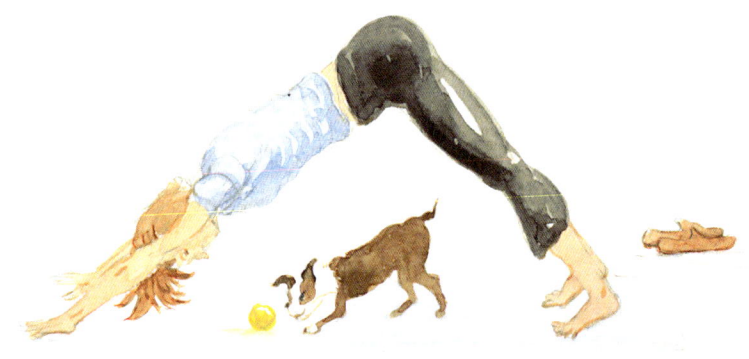

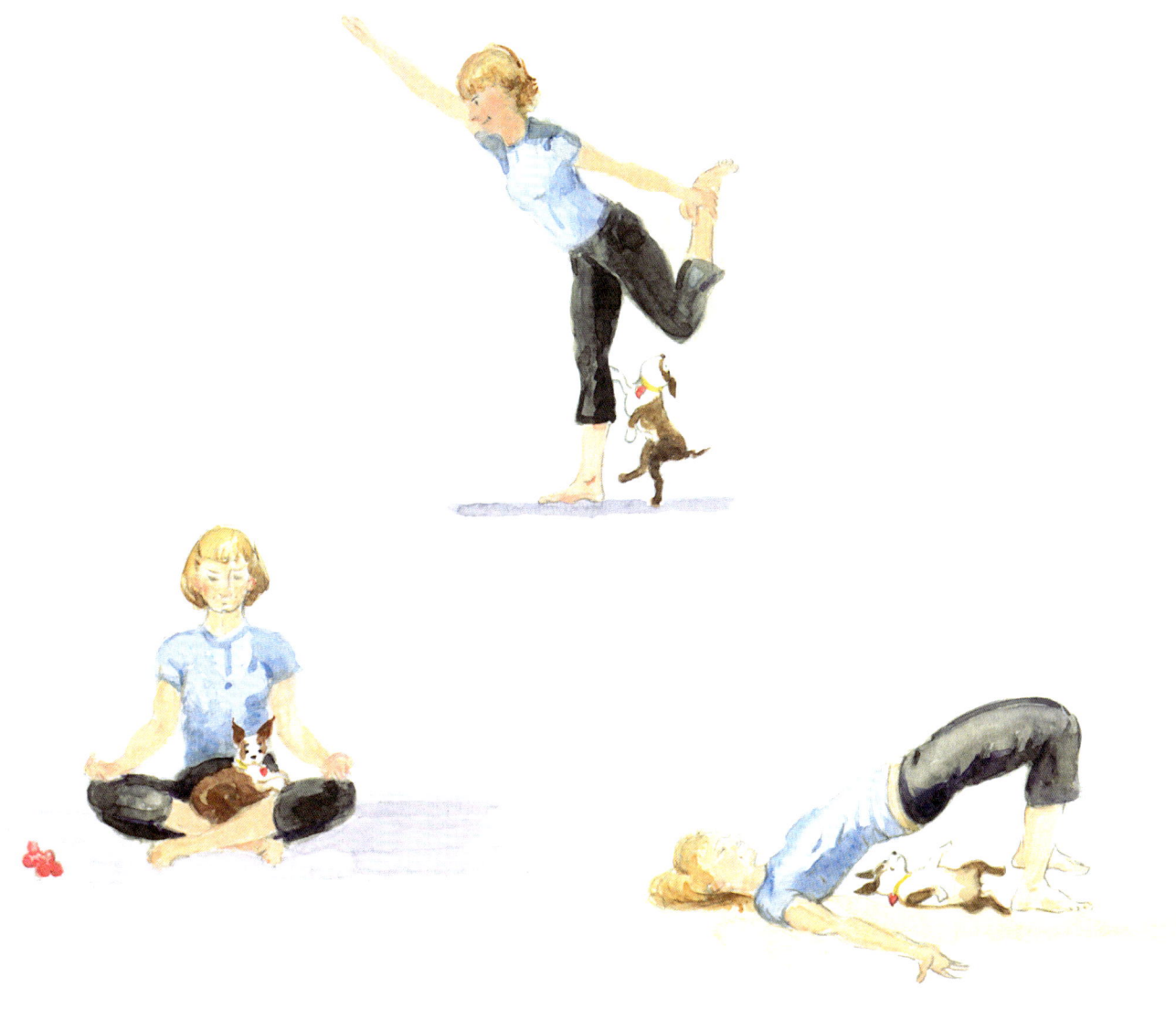

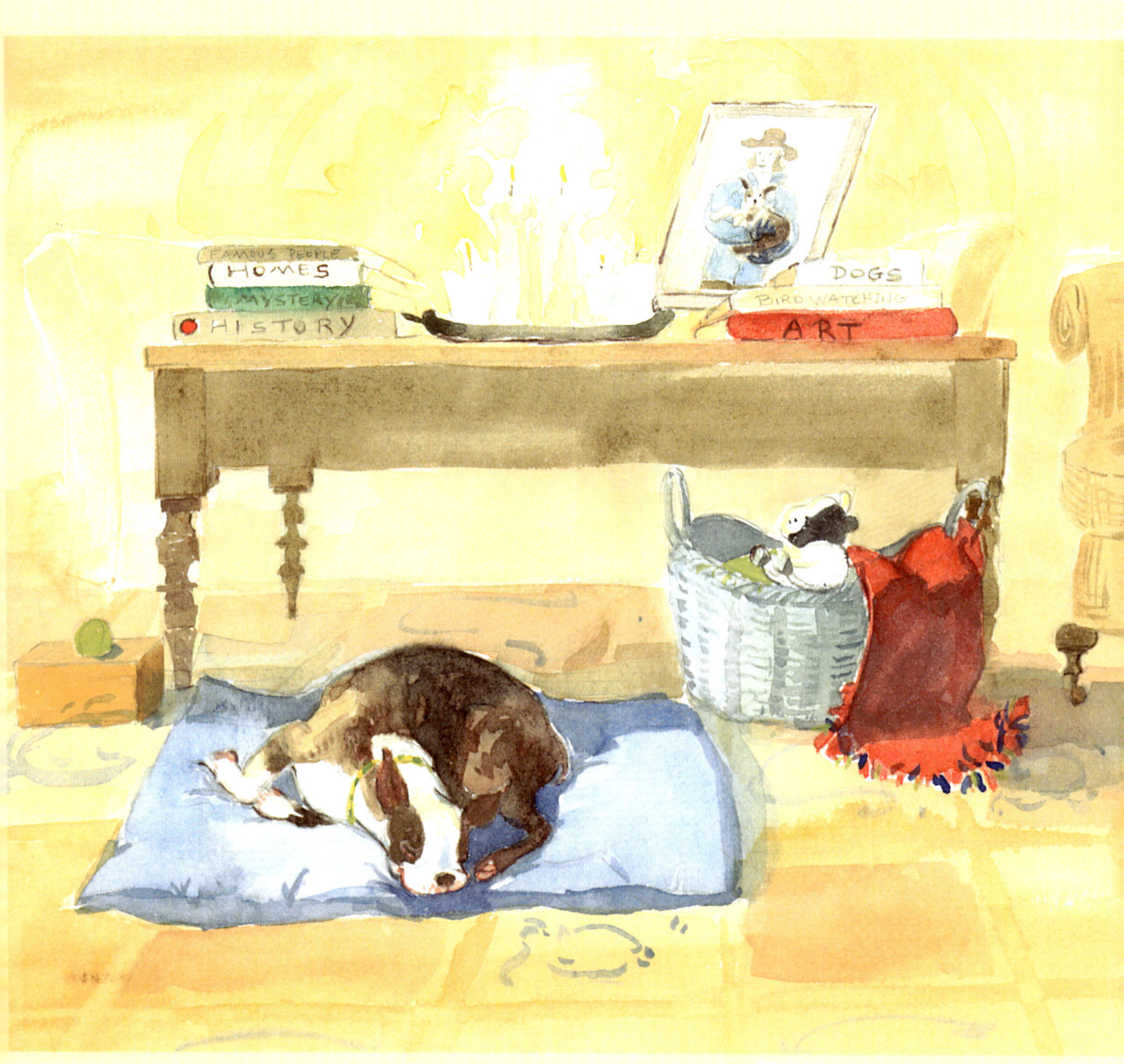

Another day went by and Sadie was feeling that same tug at her heart. She was also beginning to create some new exciting dreams.

Then someone special came along…

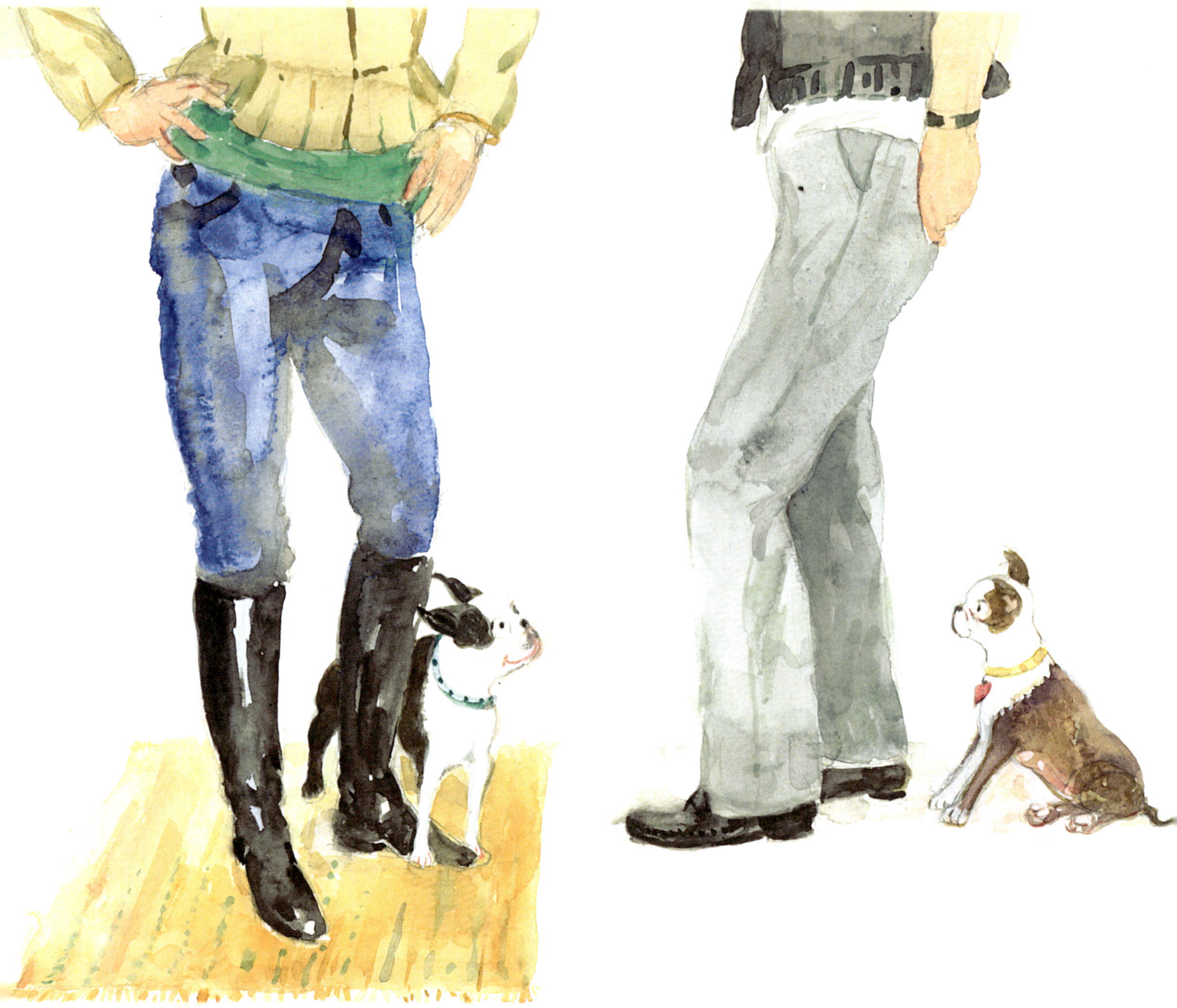

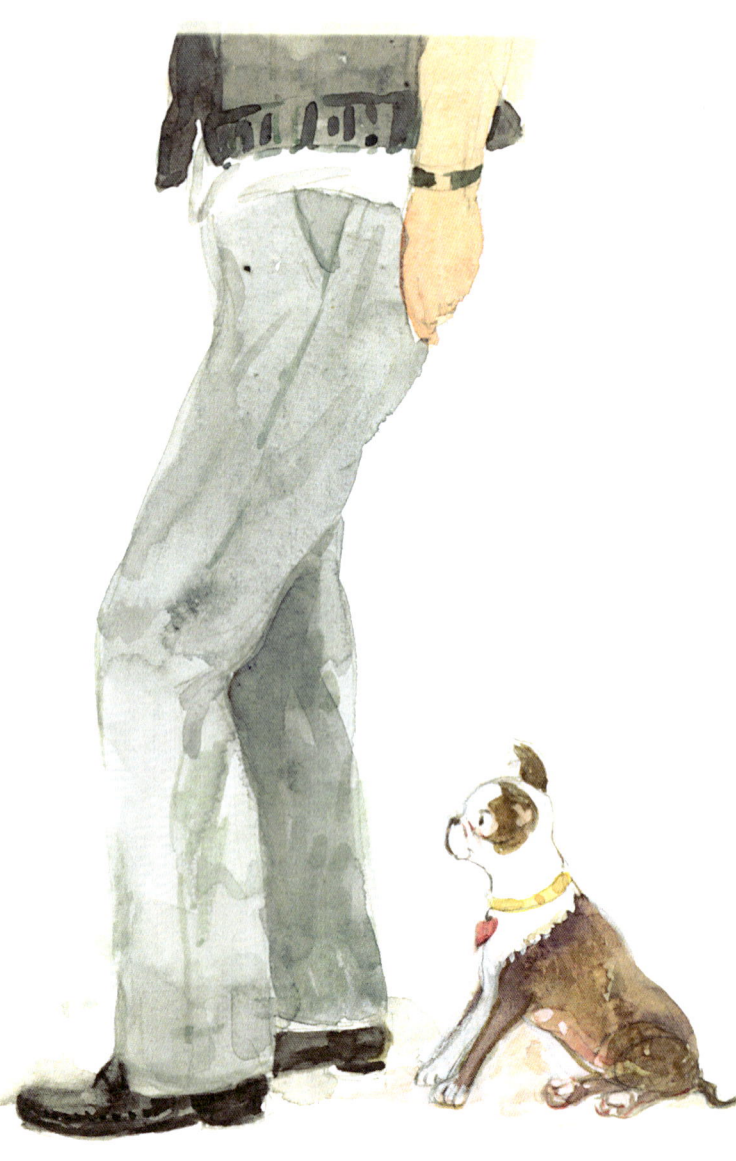

Sadie met Daysi, and she was just like her!

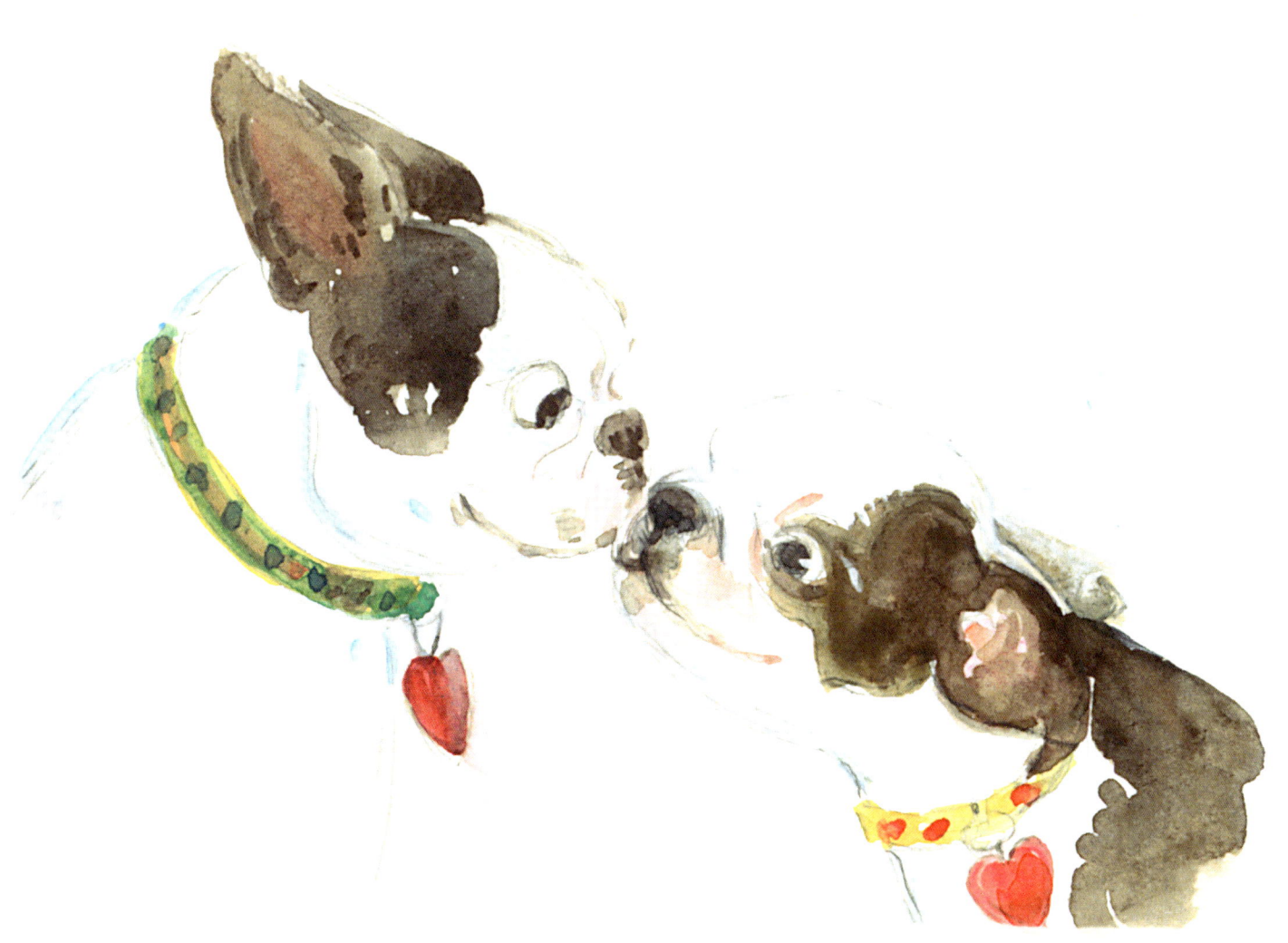

They played…

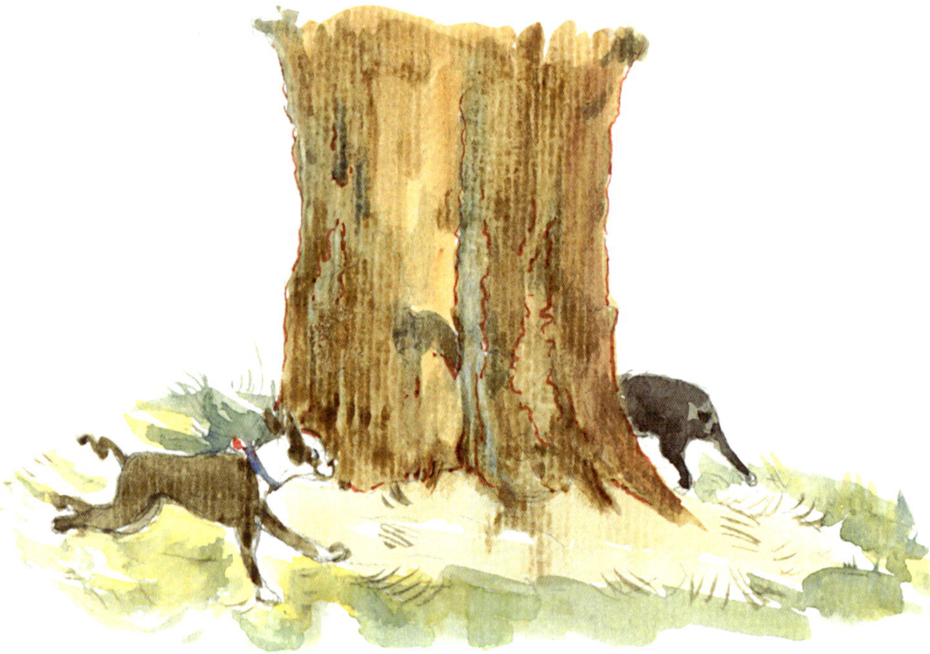

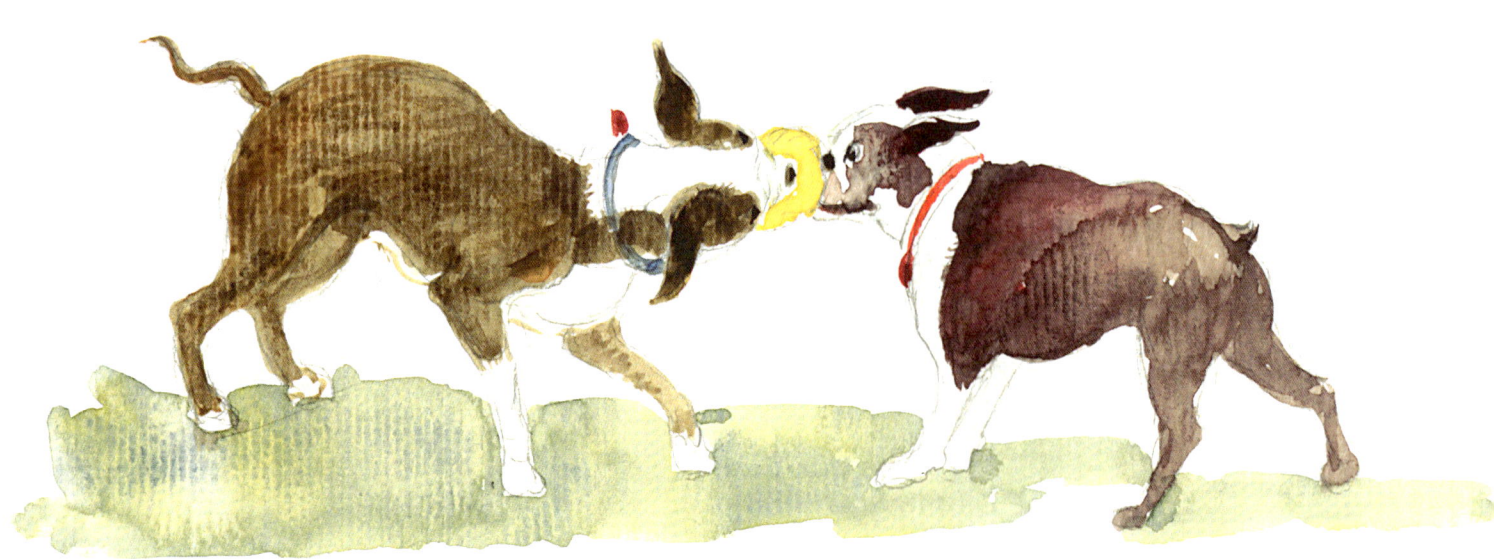

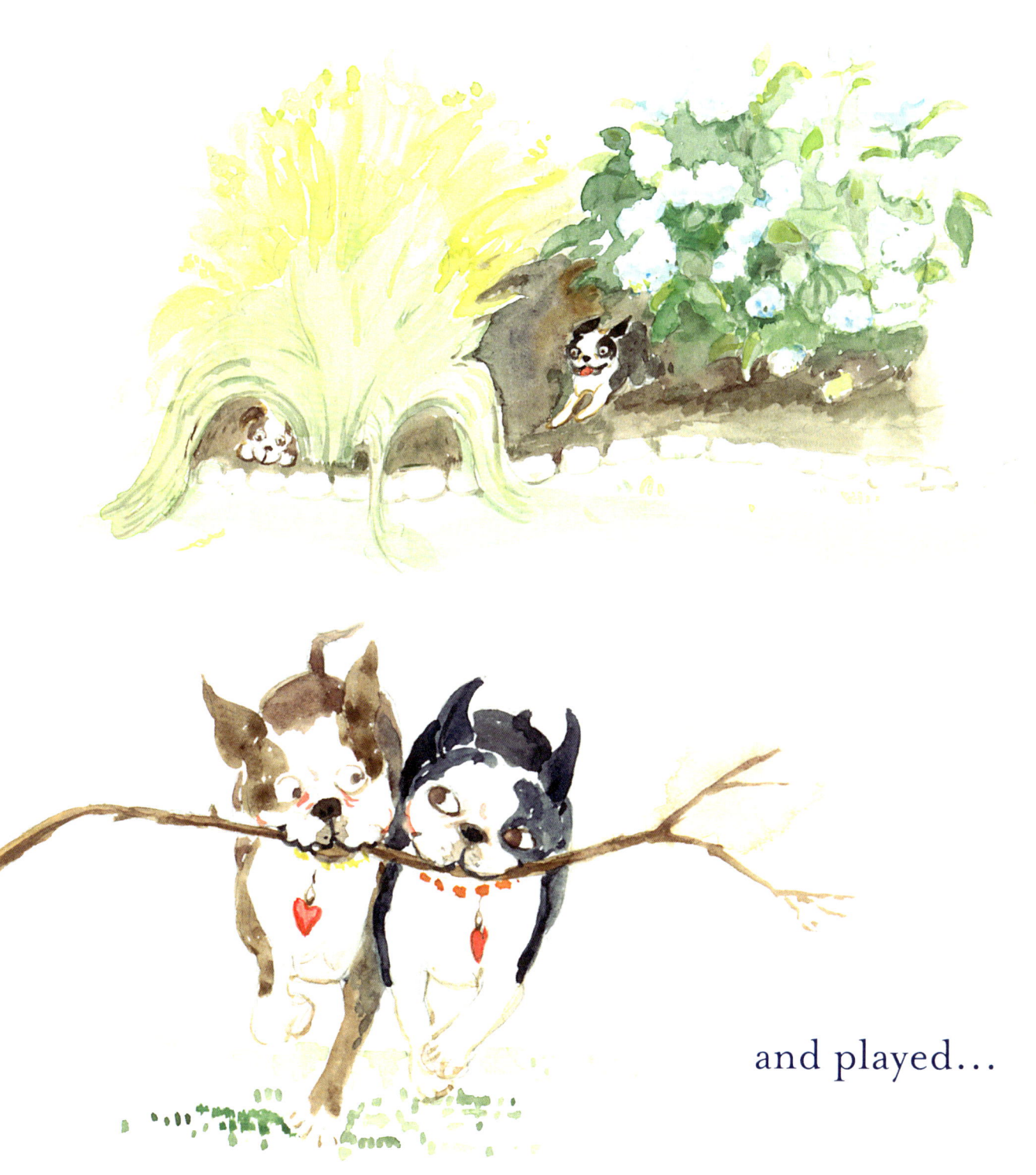

and played...

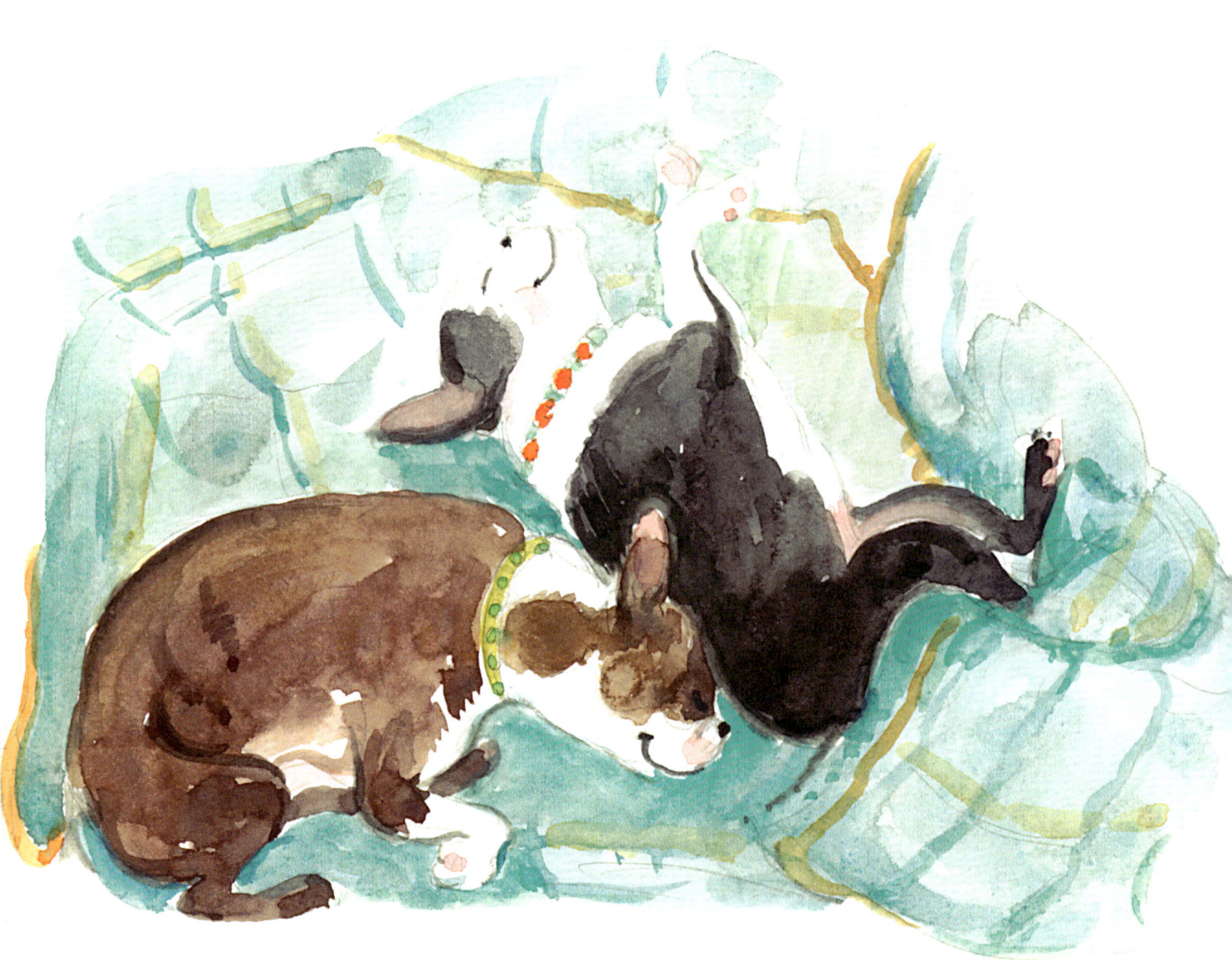

and then they happily rested.

That night Sadie was very tired and very happy. She said goodbye to Daysi and just wanted to climb into her own bed and sleep. What a good night's sleep it was too.

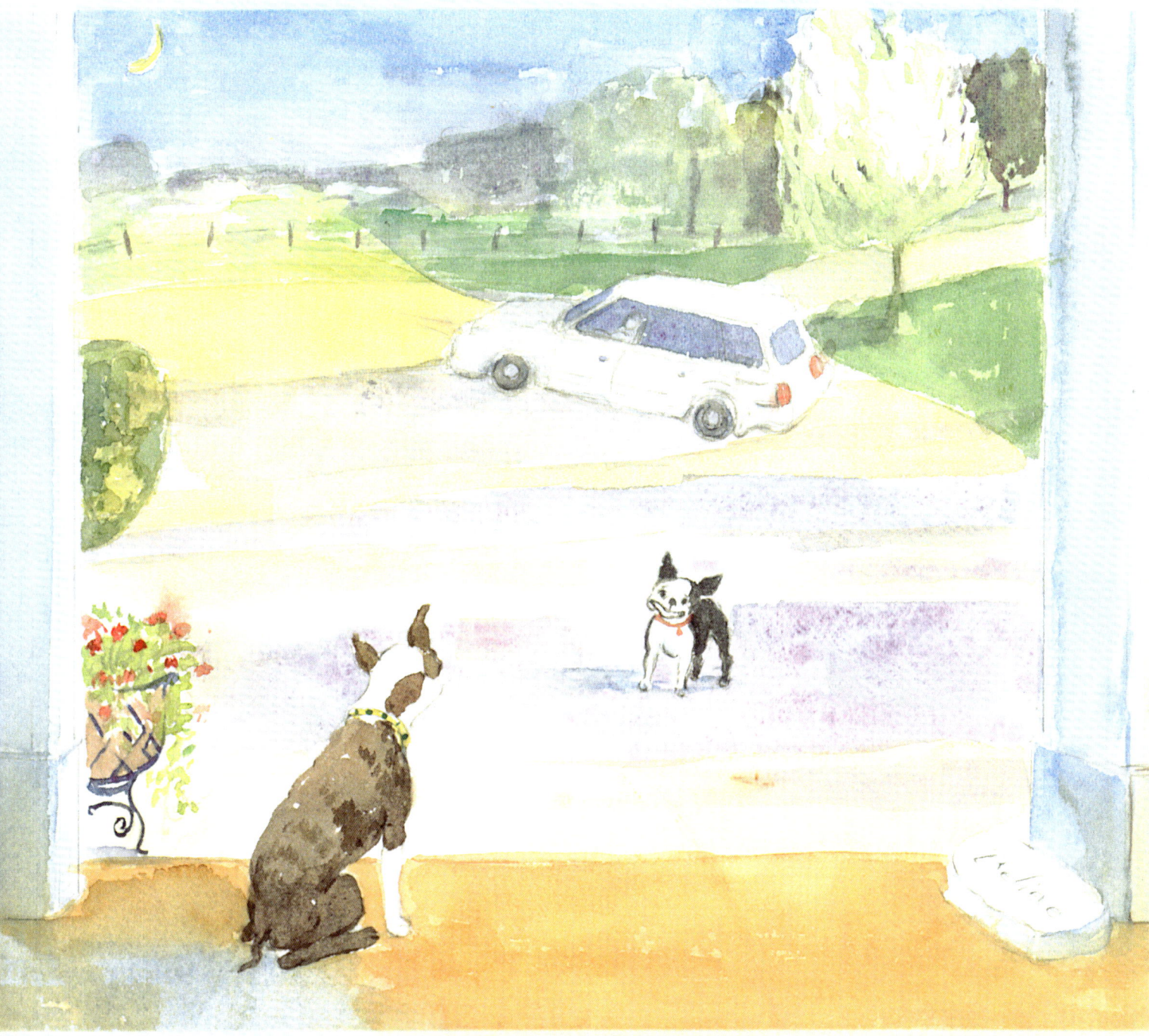

The next morning, Sadie awoke in her bed happy and with—not a small tug—but a warm, glowing feeling in her heart.

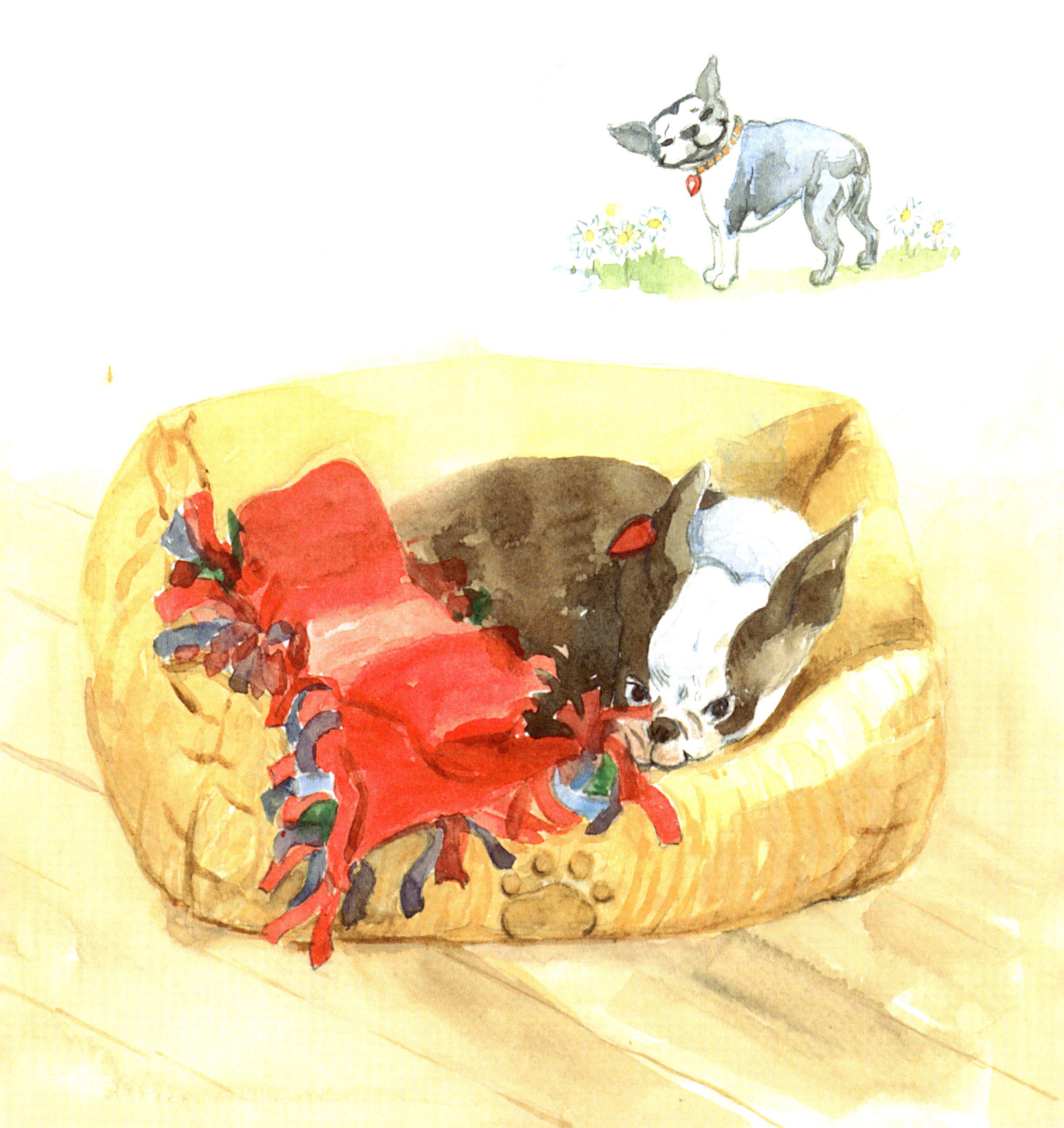

Awake now, Sadie Bug was learning that each day includes all the exciting things she found around her: sitting in her mom's comfy lap, lying next to big dog Anne, exploring her wonderful yard, and best of all, playing with her new best friend Daysi!

Having sweet dreams from now on, Sadie nestled into the warmth of her home in the country and thought of all the special friends she had now. She couldn't wait to have Daysi over for their next play day. Together they would have more adventures and visit all of Sadie's other friends.

And, best of all, she wasn't lonely anymore.

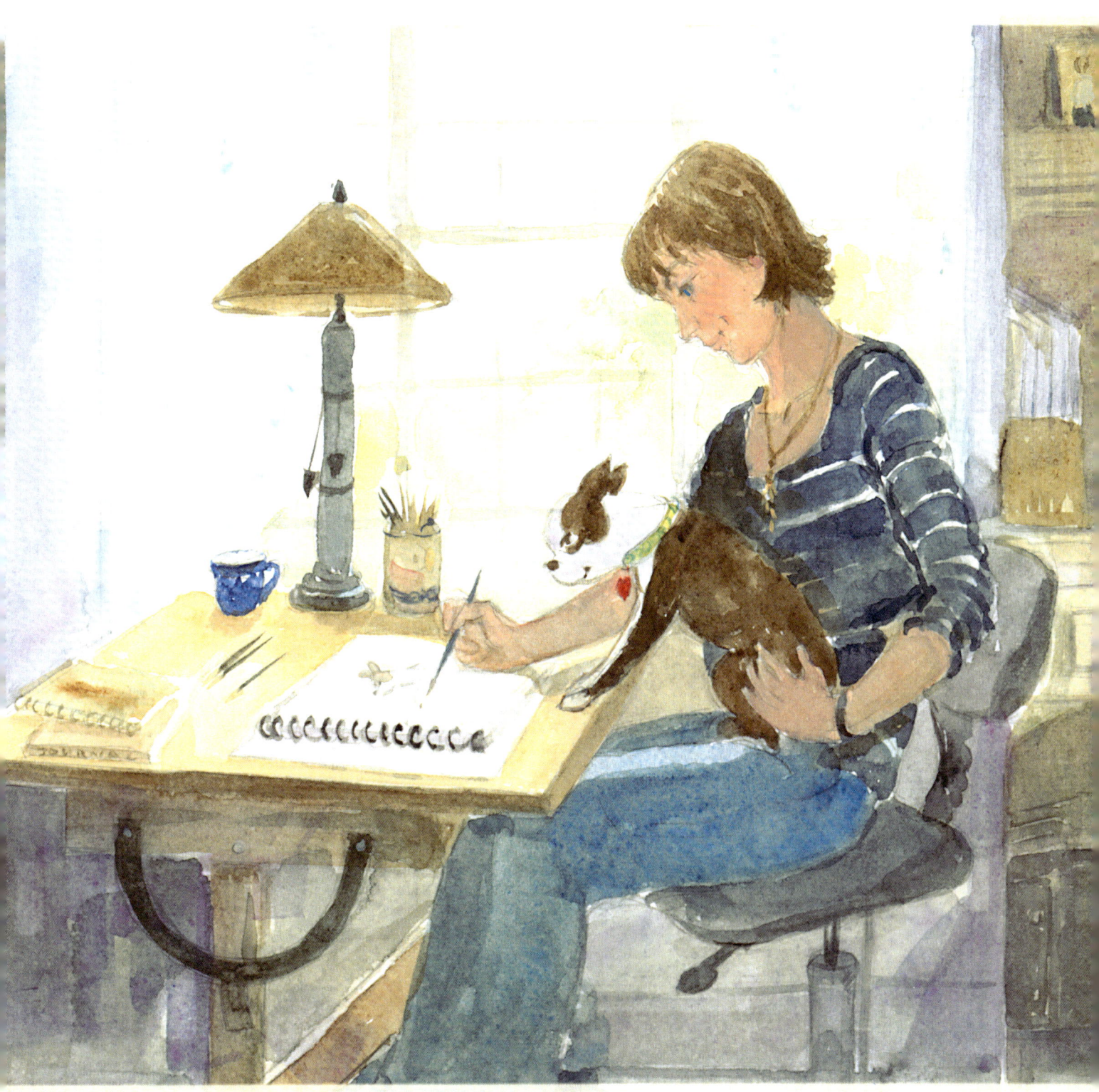

Elizabeth Brandon

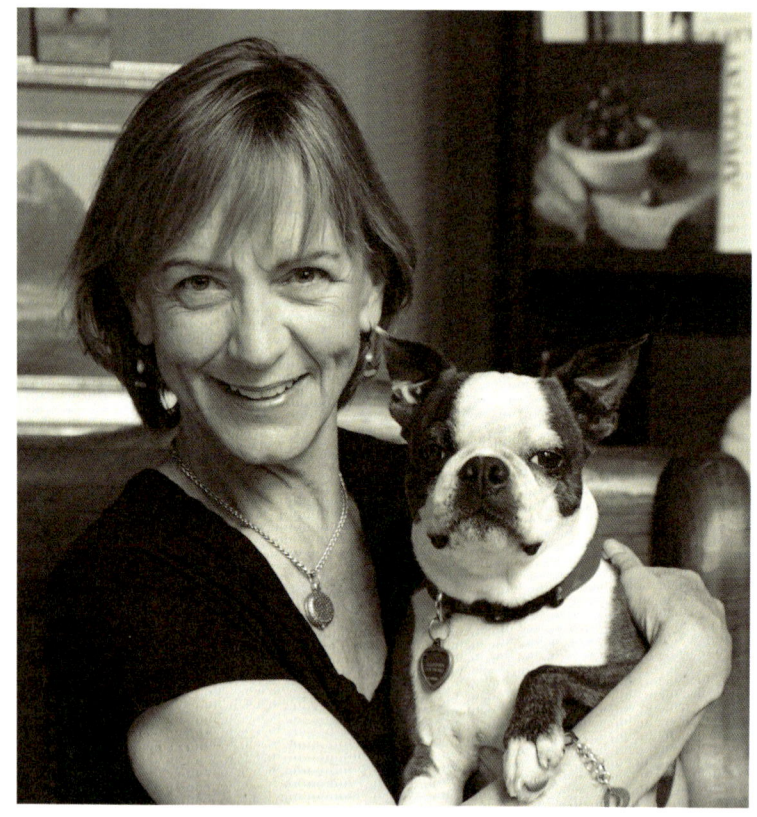

A little brindle Boston Terrier entered Elizabeth's life and the story of Sadie Bug was born. "Upon Sadie's arrival, her puppy innocence awakened my desire to share with others her sense of adventure and her loving spirit. Sadie Bug has taught me about the enormous value of the companionship and unique love of a little dog with a big heart and a funny screw tail."

Elizabeth Brandon is a classical artist following the old master tradition of Rembrandt and Frans Hals. The transient nature of light and atmosphere upon her subject inspires her to capture the living essence of still life, florals and landscapes. To learn more about the artist and her paintings, please visit www.elizabethbrandon.com

Elizabeth Brandon lives and works in middle Tennessee with her artist-husband, Joseph H Sulkowski, who shares her love of dogs. His dog and sporting art are collected worldwide.

Sadie, Daysi and Vincent play together often at their home in the country.

CPSIA information can be obtained
at www.ICGtesting.com
Printed in the USA
BVXC01n2057100615
404040BV00009B/54